STROKE DIARY

The Secret of Aphasia Recovery

STROKE DIARY

The Secret of Aphasia Recovery

Thomas G. Broussard, Jr., Ph.D.

Stroke Educator, Inc.
St. Augustine, Florida

Book and cover design by Sagaponack Books & Design

ISBN: 978-0-9979653-2-2 (softcover)
ISBN: 978-0-9979653-3-9 (e-book)
Library of Congress Catalog Card Number: 2016914173

Summary: The second book in the Stroke Diary trilogy explores and explains enriched speech therapy as the missing link between conventional speech therapy and intensive speech therapy

MED057000-MEDICAL/Neuroscience
SCI089000-SCIENCE/Life Sciences/Neuroscience

www.StrokeEducator.com

Stroke Educator, Inc.
St. Augustine, Florida

Printed and bound in USA
First Edition

To Laura,

Josiane, David and Will,

Mira, Kai, Maddie, and Jack

The world breaks everyone, and afterward, some are strong at the broken places.

—Ernest Hemingway

ar·ti·fact

ar·ti·fact \är-ti-fakt\ ***n*** [L *arte* by skill (abl. of *art-*, *ars* skill) + *factum*, neut. of *factus*, pp. of *facere* to do — more at ARM, DO] [1821] **1 a:** something created by humans usu. for a practical purpose; *esp:* an object remaining from a particular period <caves containing prehistoric *~s*> **b:** something characteristic of or resulting from a particular human institution, period, trend, or individual <self-consciousness ... turns out to be an ~ of our education system —*Times Lit. Supp.*> **2:** a product of artificial character (as in a scientific test) due usu. to extraneous (as human) agency — **ar·ti·fac·tu·al** \ är-ti-fak-che(-we)l, -fak-shwel\ ***adj***

CONTENTS

PREFACE

This book is the second of a trilogy. When I started thinking about writing a book about my stroke, writing *one* book was the goal. As I considered what one book might require, it grew into two books and then three.

The first book, *Stroke Diary: A Primer for Aphasia Therapy*, offered the facts as best I knew them. All of the data provide an almost day-to-day account of my recovery for about two years, starting with pictures I took at the hospital. I saved my calendars, my speech therapy session reports, and doctors' notes. I ordered all of the materials from Massachusetts General Hospital (MGH), from the time in the emergency room (ER) until my discharge. I asked for all the reports from my rehabilitation hospital and received the SLP, OT, and PT records.

I was lucky enough to have recorded most of the journey using my diary, recording my voice on my iPhone, and taking pictures. I couldn't read, write, or speak well. That was the rub. I *wrote* my diary with metaphorical drawings and nonsensical sentences. It took eleven months before I realized that what I *thought* was good was, in fact, bad. But the evidence, as bad as it was, was still a treasure trove of information about my metamorphosis from a pupa to a butterfly.

This book, *Stroke Diary: The Secret of Aphasia Recovery*, draws more evidence from my diary and research since then. This book provides the explanations of the *how* and the *why* of my recovery, and exposes the missing link between conventional speech therapy and intensive speech therapy. Enriched speech therapy is what is missing.

My recovery was the result of practicing more language activities and experiences. That was *how* I did it. But *why* did I do the things that needed to be done? There is more that can be done *earlier* in the therapeutic process. The brain can get better with regular, persistent, and personal intensive activities. The brain will get better with conventional speech therapy *plus* "enriched" speech therapy *delivered at the same time.*

Conventional speech therapy primes the pump. Enriched speech therapy provides a steady flow of day-to-day experience-dependent activities. The interaction of reading, writing, and speaking convert the experience of life into plasticity, the ability to alter and enhance a new mind.

Whether it is damaged or not, the brain learns every day. It is built that way. When your brain is damaged, we call it therapy. When your brain is healthy or intact, we call it learning. Yet the process of improving your brain is the same. Therapy is learning, and learning is therapy.

INTRODUCTION

The secret of recovery from aphasia isn't a secret at all. Aphasia recovery is all about *the doing*. When you have lost your language from a stroke, the best thing to do is practice your language, damaged as it is. It is both the curse and the blessing.

I had my stroke and aphasia in 2011. People with aphasia talk about "losing their language" as if that is what happened. We don't lose our *entire* language as much as we have individual modalities each with their own deficits. I could speak fairly well, read poorly, and could not write at all, all at the same time. Yet within each modality, there were additional levels of sub-routines, each with their own individual deficits. Not unlike the way we created language the first time, aphasia recovery re-creates our language in much the same way, one cell, one neuron, and one synapse at a time.

I have heard it said before that some people with aphasia won't do anything *until* they get better. Why not wait until your brain gets better on its own? It doesn't work that way. You cannot get better without exercising your damaged language. Writing, reading, and speaking are the only tools. If you don't practice, you won't do as well. It has been said many times that sharpening a saw is half the battle. The cut cuts faster if you sharpen your saw.

My speech therapy sessions were conducted twice a week, but it wasn't enough. I primed every exercise. I did my homework, but I needed more practice. My therapist recommended that I check out one of the few intensive aphasia programs in the country. I reviewed their website. The cost was very expensive and I certainly didn't have the money. But the program itself sounded a lot like practice to me, and more practice was what I needed.

I could not read, write, or speak well. More than that, I couldn't *tell* I was unaware of my deficits. Being unaware was the biggest deficit of all. Unable to read, write, or speak well was one thing. Being *unaware* of being unable to communicate was another. None of this made sense to me at the time. I used my tools before I knew they were dull. I know, it doesn't make any sense. The saw had to sharpen itself.

Our brain is the saw. The only way to sharpen it is to use it. It is the only way. There is no pill. There is no medicine. There is only practice and motivation. If practice is the engine, motivation is the key.

And not all motivation is conscious. I discovered that a number of (unconscious) steps drew me to practice my language without being consciously motivated to make those steps. In my mind were a number of synonyms, but they seemed somewhat different. When I tried to find the one word I wanted, many words flew by as I considered (reflected, thought, deliberated) what the right word would be. I used this construction (a word, plus two or three similar words) throughout this book to indicate the way my thinking presented itself as it groped for the right word or feeling.

Most of my activities were automatic, instinctive, and involuntary (in the sense of being without conscious control). They also turned out to be therapeutic. As soon as I started walking, my mind started racing. I thought every day (most people do), so I kept track of my thoughts to reexamine what I had been thinking. I couldn't examine what didn't exist without the evidence. I couldn't remember *what I didn't remember* without some physical proof of what I was thinking. I kept a diary. I recorded my voice. I took pictures. The evidence of my thinking was the first step. Feedback was the next. Evidence permitted the inexorable drive for feedback to occur. You can't have one without the other.

Exercise, evidence, feedback, and the resultant awareness were seed stock for the process of recovery. The principles of plasticity underlie the experience-dependent activities that engendered it. Every person with aphasia has the capacity to improve. *Knowing* is one of the key words. More knowing provides more knowing. However, the first step is the *doing*: regular, persistent, intensive, repeated, and varied mechanisms for action. That is the path to recovery.

Regular speech therapy is limited to the number of sessions mandated by insurance. The end of insurance coverage is the end of speech therapy and is tantamount to the end of hopeful recovery. Intensive speech therapy is also available, although it is expensive and sparse. At the end of speech therapy, most people with aphasia are left with no treatment, no therapy, and less recovery than the therapy they can afford.

There is another option. Exercise, walking, and the resultant enriched environment can provide non-prescriptive neurological benefits on your own. The more I walked, the more I thought. Walking triggered other activities with therapeutic benefits far beyond speech therapy. Problem solving, metaphor making, evidence providing, feedback shaping, and awareness creating formed the basis for a new, enriched therapeutic environment.

STROKE DIARY

The Secret of Aphasia Recovery

Part 1

Initial Steps to Recovery

CHAPTER ONE
SPEECH THERAPY

We discovered that education is not something which the teacher does, but that it is a natural process which develops spontaneously in the human being.

—Maria Montessori

I met my speech-language pathologist at Newton-Wellesley Hospital in Newton, Massachusetts, for my assessment. She was a bright, energetic woman. I was happy to meet her. It had been a month since my stroke and I still didn't know where I stood with my problems. My daughter had helped me, as did my wife. But I still couldn't tell what was *really* wrong. And I still had no idea how I could get better. You can only imagine what it feels like when your language is "broken." How do you fix that when you can't tell it's damaged?

When I was young, I broke my hand (from football). I could feel the pain. My hand was swollen. I could point out the exact place (center bone) where I had been kicked. As a result of my stroke, I could not give rise to what had happened. There was no pain. There were no symptoms that I could see. There was no consciousness that I was conscious of. I was walking across the street and felt a "click" in my brain. It felt like the sound of a switch. I froze, staring at my foot. From that point on, I couldn't explain anything. My brain was injured: the explanations *themselves* were the things that were broken. If this was a disease, it wasn't something that felt bad. The weather was nice. The sun was beautiful. The air was crisp and cool. It was a wonderful day, and I felt fine. I couldn't understand why I wasn't fine. It was like waiting to hear from your doctor about your recent tests. I felt fine because I *was* fine. I had no other reason to think otherwise.

I had an appointment with my therapist the week after the assessment. If there were any real problems, the assessment would highlight them. My therapist used several paper-and-pencil tests, including the Boston Diagnostic Aphasia Examination (BDAE) and the Boston Naming Test (BNT). I was eager to get started. I felt as if something was wrong, but I couldn't put my finger on it. It had been almost a month since my stroke and the physical symptoms were getting better. I was sleeping better and eating better. Everything was getting better and the assessment was the icing on the cake. If I still had some remaining problems, they couldn't be that bad. It could have been a "minor" case of aphasia.

My assessment took about an hour and a half. The test looked a lot like the old SAT tests. It included verbal expression, written expression, auditory comprehension, and reading comprehension. I went through them quickly. I really didn't know whether I was going fast or slow. I couldn't remember if I was making mistakes or not. In tests at school, I was usually aware if I was making a mistake. In the speech assessment, I didn't notice any errors per se. As a result, I thought I had done well. I thought I would be discharged after the test, without any real problems.

After the assessment, the therapist recommended that we arrange additional sessions. I knew I'd have to come back to get the results. I didn't realize that the words "additional sessions" were a clue to what was to come.

We met again and I got the report. It turned out that I could only read single words and short sentences. I read the entire report, but couldn't fully grasp what it meant. As the report said: "Short paragraph comprehension with 70% accuracy and *complete breakdown at lengthy paragraph level (beyond 5 sentences).*"

My therapist understood I had aphasia and she knew it even before my assessment. She could tell by the flaws in my spoken language. She could also tell I was aware (at least at some level) about my deficits. How *unaware* was I of my deficits? I was aware in a general way about the problems with my language. But I was unable to internalize the impact of the report. My therapist could tell I was making mistakes, but I couldn't. I was unaware that I couldn't tell I was making the errors. It wasn't the way it was in school before my stroke. Then I *knew* when I had made mistakes. I could fix them on the fly. It seemed that this particular skill was one of the many deficits yet to be identified. I couldn't tell what I couldn't tell.

I was *unaware* of being unaware. It was one of the big problems. It felt like I was in a fog. I was aware of most of my conversations with my family, friends, and therapist. The problem was that my memory appeared to be short-term and only "in the moment." What I mean is that when my therapist and I had a conversation, I understood what she meant and she understood what I meant. We would go back and forth with ideas, problems, and directions. As my therapist talked about my problems, I understood, but only "in the moment." I didn't realize that I gave the appearance of "knowing" (and gave the appearance by responding in kind), but I didn't retain "knowing" for more than a minute or two. I don't know if my therapist ever understood that while I was responding in kind, she thought I had retained the conversation, when in fact I didn't retain the knowledge for more than a few minutes. As a result, this was the "fog" of being unaware of being unaware.

I worked hard during my time with my therapist. I got better—although I still remembered things but only "in the moment." Later I realized that the time of the "in the moment" moment expanded as I got better.

The problem wasn't one definition for each deficit. It wasn't a memory thing. It wasn't a comprehension thing. It wasn't an attention thing. It was all of those things. Each deficit and sub-routines of the deficit were stimulated in different ways. Of course, at the time, I was incapable of explaining this phenomenon to anyone else. I never knew if my therapist understood this. She wrote in her report that I was "aware of my deficits." So, *she* was aware *I* was aware (at least in *my* universe), such that she recorded my performance as "getting better," as far as she knew. Whether I knew it or not, I *was* getting better, notwithstanding my short-term memory deficits.

After the first session, I asked if I could have copies of her reports. I read them over and over. At the time, they still didn't mean a lot to me. The more reports I had, the more I could "read" the evidence. As weeks went by, I could see I was getting better as evidenced by my therapist's perspective in her report. Each report provided an objective set of scores for different exercises. The goals were adjusted upwards as I improved. Here are some of the goals.

- "Follow 3 step/complex commands with 90% accuracy" as a goal, <u>went from 50% to 80% accuracy</u>.
- "Name common object with 90% accuracy" as a goal, <u>went from 60% to 100%</u>.

- "Answer complex yes/no questions with 90% accuracy" as a goal, went from 80% to 100%.

I was beginning to realize there were two minds with different opinions of my improvement. As time went by, I could understand the reports. My "scores" were going up. That was a good thing. I could tell the scores were only part of the story. As I read the report I could see other perspectives of the same deficits that weren't part of the scores. I could do well on the goals listed above.

Even so, other indications of deficits didn't show up in my report. They didn't appear because there weren't any exercises that would tell me my grammar was gone. There were very few tests (none I knew of) that would have asked me to write a full sentence spontaneously and by hand. All of my exercises were fill-in-the-blank, lists, following directions, drawing a line, writing an X, completing a sentence, and answering complex Yes/No questions. Rewriting a sentence to correct a single error was still easy compared to spontaneous writing. It provided almost all the context of the sentence, allowing me to "see" and fix the only error.

As I reviewed the therapy reports on my own, I could tell something was amiss, given that my objective scores kept going up yet my ability to write with meaning wasn't going anywhere. As I wrote my sentence exercises (the bane of my existence!), there were still no freehand sentences. The exercise was structured with: "He is fill-in-the-blank. He is skating, he is listening, or he is driving."

Most complex sentences were written by me at home, in my computer, and emailed to my therapist. It is almost impossible to write words that are purposely wrong in a computer. "Auto-correct" in the computer was part of the reason. Neither one of us (my wife nor I) were willing to submit my sentences if they were wrong. My wife helped (offered, encouraged, cued, suggested, and I rewrote) until they looked fine. So, most of the time my sentences gave the appearance of looking right. There were a few times at the therapist's office when my sentences didn't look so good. The therapist sat me at the computer and had me write some of my own sentences. Sorry to say, my scores went up or down depending on whether I was home (with help) or at the therapist's office (without help). I learned later what "max cue" meant. "Max cue" basically means that someone else did (almost all of) my work. Many people "help" in that regard: therapists, professional staff, volunteers, family, and friends. Socially, it helps, but it doesn't really "help" in the larger scheme.

The overarching context of my language was still the problem. We were both working on the same goal from two different perspectives. My therapist was coming from the bottom up. Individual words, lists, simple tasks, command tasks, and simple sentences were the measureable scores of performance. At the end of the day (and at the end of my therapy), my scores were going up and my performance was improving. From my perspective and the evidence from my own hand, I still couldn't write well (handwriting). I could update my résumé, make an application, or write a cover letter with my computer (with a month full of Sundays). But I couldn't write a handwritten thank-you note.

I had never shown my diary to my therapist (or anyone else). I wonder what would have happened if the two worlds had collided? I was asked that question at a presentation. If I had shown my diary to the therapist, it was possible it would have been a shortcut to recovery. If I had actually *seen* the mistakes, which is to say if I had the self-awareness of the errors *at that moment* to *see* them, that was one thing. Who knows? Would my awareness have appeared spontaneously? That would have been magical. But it was what it was. It was an experiment. I would have ruined the experiment if I had announced what I otherwise couldn't announce.

CHAPTER TWO
MOTIVATION

When we are no longer able to change a situation, we are challenged to change ourselves.

—Viktor E. Frankl
Man's Search for Meaning

I have always had a general sense of being motivated. As a result, I often accomplished much of what I wanted. But for many years, I didn't consciously study the unconscious part of my mind. As I got older I became more conscious of the mental effort of setting and achieving goals. At a certain point, I was aware of these behaviors. Of course, I acted on the practice long before I was *aware* of the activity—otherwise called a routine or habit.

I imagine "motivation" was drilled into me (usually in good ways) by my father. As I recognized my habits, I started remembering motivational stories about my father. Motivational stories from my dad usually included some amount of anxiety and fear. I kept tabs on these stories, and only recently asked my kids if I had been "motivating" them in similar ways. I would like to say the jury is still out, but I could see it in their eyes. They remember being motivated, and to me, that is a good thing.

I tried to remember the earliest motivational story from my dad. Locations placed in time helped solidify the memories. We lived in one house until I was eight years old, and moved to another house until my high school graduation. So it was easy to divide my memories between Paoli, Pennsylvania, and Wayne, Pennsylvania, a few miles away. As a result, I had only a few notable (and *usually* real) memories from Paoli. There were quite a few made-up memories along the way too. I used them against my siblings at Thanksgiving dinners!

It is hard to find memories when you are so young. There were good memories in Paoli, but not so much with a motivating twist. Motivational stories started after moving to Wayne.

I was in Catholic schools in Paoli. We moved to public schools in Wayne during the summer after my third-grade year. Immediately there were problems. My birthday is January 25. I was young for my grade in Paoli. When we moved, the new school had a fall cutoff date (I don't remember … September, October?) for matriculation. My parents went to the school to see the principal. They brought me with them. They were talking. I was just a kid. I imagine I probably wasn't listening. I sat there and read a book (I always read books).

At a certain point, my dad invited me into the conversation. He told me there was a problem. Because of my age, the school wanted me to "stay back" and do third grade again. My parents wanted me to go into fourth grade. Apparently, my parents got heated enough that the principal agreed if I would agree. My father explained the situation. He said I was young and if I stayed in the third grade, I would "stay back." If I moved into the fourth grade, I would be "ahead." I don't really remember the exact conversation. Basically, they said it was up to me. So I agreed. I must have liked the idea of being "ahead"! As the years went by, I remembered the story because I had heard it so many times.

The rest was history. I was 16 years old for most of my senior year. I was admitted to the US Naval Academy (USNA) when I was just 17. That story was the beginning of memories with motivational lessons from my dad.

It turned out that many motivational stories came from my father. I loved baseball and was a pitcher in the Tiger League (and then the Babe Ruth League). I was a decent batter too. We had to sell tickets for a raffle every year to raise money for the league. As I remember it, we sold tickets for a quarter each and five tickets for a dollar. There was always a big prize for the player who sold the most tickets. In one particular year, the prize was a MacGregor baseball glove. The glove was placed in a glass cabinet with a spotlight shining on it. To me, it appeared like King Arthur's sword. I wanted that glove! I got my allotted tickets and went to Dad and asked what I should do. I told him I wanted the glove badly. He said I should sell as many tickets as possible. I started selling tickets that weekend and sold all of them that week. So I asked Dad again what else I could do. He said I should find out how many tickets had been sold last year, and try to sell more than that. I found out that about 375 tickets had been sold (by the winner) the year before. I got another allotment of tickets and sold them all. There were still several weeks to go in the campaign, so I asked Dad again. I had sold the same amount as last year—375 tickets. I was worried, and desperate about winning "my" glove. It would be awful if one player sold just one more ticket than I did. My dad told me if I sold double the amount of tickets, I would probably win. As I said, there was still plenty of time, so I doubled the goal again and sold a total of 750 tickets. We lived in a small town, so I was able to walk into the center of town and sell tickets to all the merchants. By then, they knew who I was. After I had sold 750 tickets, there was still time left, and I was still worried. I asked Dad one more time. He told me if I doubled it again, that would be it. With two weeks left to go, I sold another 750 tickets. With over 1,500 tickets sold, I waited for the fateful day of the Little League Fundraiser Dinner in the basement of the bank in town. The glass cabinet was displayed there with my *Excalibur*.

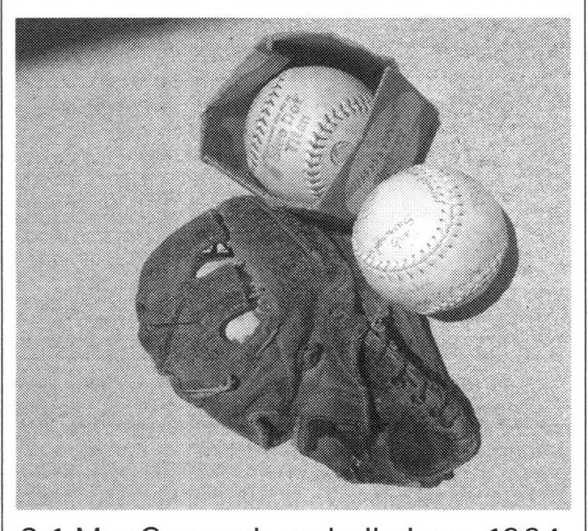

2-1 MacGregor baseball glove, 1964.

I won the MacGregor glove (figure 2-1). I found out the second-place ticket seller had sold fewer tickets than the winner from the year before. I used that mitt all my life in baseball and softball leagues and in work leagues (I still have it.) (figure 2-2). My glove meant everything to me. It represented so much more than just baseball.

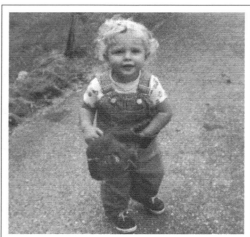

2-2 Same glove, 35 years ago with my 1½-year-old daughter.

The local bank and businesses sponsored the league. The local newspaper printed small articles (just a few lines) about every Little League game during the season. I saved every article. It was fun. Our names were there and often with a picture of the team. Probably the most important article for me was winning a game I pitched *and* also hitting a grand slam home run to win the game. It was pretty amazing, and I never did it again.

At the same time as I was playing league baseball, I decided I wanted to attend the US Naval Academy. I wanted to go to sea. I had wanted to go since the fourth grade. So, starting in junior high, I worked on the application with my dad. In those days (and probably even today), it takes time to be considered and selected to the Academy. We worked through it all. We were ready by my junior year. We met with the local US congressman. We submitted the application. We met with a USNA alumnus from the area. The only things left to do were to submit my final grades at the end of my junior year and have a physical exam at a naval hospital. At that point, we had done everything we could to be considered.

Then Dad died.

He died the day after my 16th birthday. Dad looked like me, tall and thin. Dad had high blood pressure and cholesterol problems (I didn't know I would have the same later). He died of a heart attack. It was on a Friday night. There was a dance that night at school, but I didn't go because we were decorating our house for a surprise party the next night for our parents' 20th wedding anniversary. Somehow the word got to the dance that my dad had died. My dad was young, 49 years old. So, most of my friends had never experienced the death of a parent before. Many kids showed up at the house that night, just to be there with us.

Dad's funeral was a couple of days later. Before they closed his casket, I added the home run article in his pocket.

It has been in his pocket ever since. Before Dad's death, I had often thought about making a copy of it. Copiers were hard to come by and home copiers didn't even exist. But the article has always been there. It felt like a good omen. I didn't realize it still had plenty of power.

Dad had done everything he could to make sure we were ready for the USNA selection. My final grades for 11th grade went in (and they weren't all that good). That winter a friend of my dad's took me to the Philadelphia Naval Hospital at the shipyard for my physical examination. That was it. Then I waited.

It turned out my appointment type was a "competitive" appointment. Ten young men (women started four years after me) were considered as possible candidates. Each of us had to go through the application. Out of the ten, six of us were considered "qualified." One of the six qualified candidates got the appointment. I was considered "qualified," although I didn't know where I stood in the ranking. But someone "above me" got the appointment.

That was the end of it, as far as I knew. Then I got the word of other types of appointments: Since I was still "qualified," I would go into another pool. It turned out, after all of the competitive appointments had been taken, the Secretary of the Navy would fill up the class to the right manpower strength. What was called the SECNAV Qualified Candidate Pool was used for that purpose. I was put into that pool.

I had been told that the school used something called "whole man" criteria for selection. I got points for everything in my portfolio: academics, sports, community, student government, finances, and so on. It was rationalized at 100. Months went by without any news. I had applied to other schools as well. Then we just waited.

Eventually my mom had to sell our home and move to a smaller place. Mom had always taken care of the four kids full-time, but after Dad died she had to get a job. I was accepted at Penn State and figured I would go there. I graduated from high school on June 8, 1969. State College, PA. here we come.

And the following week, I received a letter stating I had been accepted to the Academy. I had to arrive by June 30, 1969. I had been selected as a SECNAV Qualified Candidate. How did it happen? We had done everything we could. It wasn't until years later that I realized my dad's motivational stories still had power.

I must have gotten one more point in my ranking for the "whole man" equation. I was sure I got credit from Dad's death and the financial burden of a widow with four young children. That must have provided the final impetus.

Relative to present-day motivations, my therapist had written in my prognosis: "Excellent, given family support, pt. motivation, young age, intelligence and awareness of deficit." She had said more than once I was "motivated." I was not aware of being *conscious* of participating in any motivational act. It did appear motivation was part of my habit.

Many books about aphasia cover the topic and the problems of motivation. Basically, the researchers state that most people who were motivated *after* their stroke were motivated based on being motivated *before* their stroke.

For many years before my stroke, I was in a position of responsibility. I can recall times when some people were *not* motivated. It was always difficult to *make* them motivated. There were plenty of people within my staff who were motivated, so I was lucky enough to have hired them "built" that way. Hiring someone who is talented but unmotivated is a thorny problem. If they were talented, they must have been motivated at some point. If they were unmotivated, it would take more (sometimes a lot more) effort to help them "get better," as it were.

My speech therapist often said she wished there was a pill for motivation. Recovery from aphasia is a difficult problem. According to scientists, researchers, and speech therapists, the first step of recovery is motivation. How do you take the first step to recovery *without* motivation? That is the problem.

In my lifetime I have read a lot about leadership, management, and teamwork. Motivation was a large part of it. I understood motivation from my perspective; I knew what motivation meant to me. When I worked with people who didn't appear motivated, it seemed like more of an angry attitude of not *wanting* to do what had to be done. I didn't know if there was a "mechanism' by which motivation could be activated (encouraged, triggered, initiated).

How does motivation occur? Is there a trigger? I knew what motivation was when I saw it. It was hard to change it in someone else's mind and body. I think motivation is a habit or a routine operating unconsciously on a day-to-day basis.

I built motivational genes by virtue of life experiences with my dad and others. I didn't think about it day-to-day until there was a need—like a 911 event in your brain. It was an "all hands on deck" emergency which required motivation first and foremost.

After my stroke, I had been reading about the brain, cell networks, and something called *plasticity*. Plasticity led me to *The Principles of Psychology* by William James. I had never heard of it before. It is a 1,200-page document, so you can't be fainthearted. It is so big I had to copy each chapter and take each one with me everywhere I went. I started reading it two years ago and I am still not halfway through it. I did read

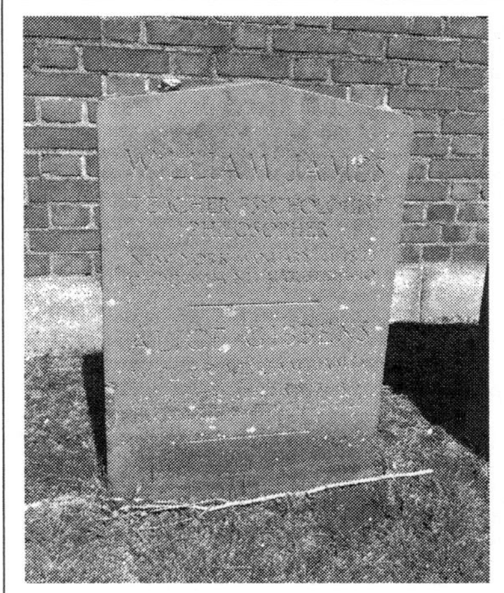

2-3 James' grave, Cambridge Cemetery, Cambridge, MA.

every chapter that discussed plasticity. Plasticity appeared in many chapters, from different perspectives. James talked about habit, will, attention, and effort, and plasticity in chapter 4, *Habit*. After reading about James and his thoughts about the brain, I was so excited I went to see his grave in Cambridge, Massachusetts (figure 2-3). This is an excerpt from the chapter on *Habit*.

> *So nothing is easier than to imagine how, when a current once traversed a path, it should traverse it more readily still a second time. But what made it ever traverse it the first time?* (James, 109)

How do you start the process of recovery? There is only one way: motivation and practice. That is all there is. Practice is easy when motivation is in charge. Without motivation, practice is in idle gear. If you don't want to take the first step, recovery becomes a problem. How do you become "motivated" when you weren't motivated before? You have to connect the dots of motivational experiences at some earlier points in your life. Or create an environment allowing motivation to grow.

Or as James said:

> *We cannot say the will, for, though many, perhaps most, human habits were once voluntary actions, no action, as we shall see in a later chapter, can be primarily such. While an habitual action may once have been voluntary, the voluntary action must before that, at least once, have been impulsive or reflex. It is*

> *this very first occurrence of all that we consider in the text.* (James, 109)

As James said, there had to have been a first "first step" before it became a habit. In the case of people with aphasia who are *not* motivated (and therefore having difficulty with recovery), *some* setting, *some* stage, or *some* environment must be arranged such that an impulsive or reflex act can be encouraged to take the first step even if we are unaware of it. In my case, there were conscious (and unconscious) motivational paths. In the absence of *conscious* motivation, exercise and walking can provide more conscious *thinking. More* thinking can collect the isolated molecules of motivation into something tangible.

> *The only thing they can do, in short, is to deepen old paths or to make new ones; and the whole plasticity of the brain sums itself up in two words when we call it an organ in which currents pouring in from the sense-organs make with extreme facility paths which do not easily disappear.* (James, 107)

It is all about the brain. I knew I *had* a brain. I knew I was fairly good at using it. But I still didn't consider real, physical, identifiable steps (in my brain) to get (operate, drive, maneuver) from one place to another.

As James said, the brain builds deep canyons of thoughts and memories. Once done, they are difficult to erase. I couldn't forget the motivational lessons of my past which enabled my future. My future wouldn't be, without a past to consider. Motivation was the first step in understanding how my recovery could be reclaimed.

CHAPTER THREE

PRACTICE: SPEAKING, LISTENING, READING, WRITING

An ounce of practice is generally worth more than a ton of theory.

—E. F. (Ernst F.) Schumacher
Small Is Beautiful: Economics as if People Mattered

The five steps to aphasia recovery are: motivation, and practice, practice, practice, and more practice! No one had told me what it would take for me to recover. No one had told me that practice was the key. No one had told me *more* practice would result with *more* improvement. It was my habit to practice reading, writing, and speaking *before* my stroke. Practicing my language *after* my stroke was as much part of my nature as it had been previously.

The only difference was that I was now unaware of the errors I was incurring since the stroke. That was a big difference. Without my worrying about the awareness issue (since I was unaware), my habit took over. I continued using a wide range of exercises. I practiced speech therapy and homework for two hours a week. I spent the rest of my time thinking about (and practicing) how to improve my language problems. As I have said, it was my nature to do this. I didn't appreciate it yet. It was the ultimate Rorschach inkblot test. I *understood* what I was thinking, without being able to *express* my thinking to others.

Speaking

As far as I knew, I didn't speak for several days after my stroke. However, from what I have heard from others, apparently I *did* speak, just not very well.

My wife, Laura, and I were walking in the street when it happened and she asked me immediately if I was having a stroke. By then, my stroke was well on its way to breaking down my speech. I was completely dazed. I was not *unconscious*. My body was moving, but I wasn't completely conscious either. Laura told me I had tried to say something, but it didn't make any sense to her.

It took about one hour for me to get to the hospital. Once I was there, I was moved from one machine (MRI, CT scan, EEG) to another. They had to check to see what kind of stroke I had and what kind of treatment I might receive. After the doctors decided I had an ischemia stroke within the time deadline required, I was ready for tPA. The hospital protocol for tPA states the drug must be administered within three hours after a stroke. tPA dissolves the clot and prevents the damage from getting worse. The nurse gave me the drug and I (apparently) starting talking immediately. Not that I knew what I was saying. As the nurse gave me the drug, I could hear a lot of noise in my head, like popcorn popping. I could hear it! I patted my left temple and started talking like crazy. My wife and the nurse were the only people in the room. They must have appreciated that *something* was going on. The nurse made notes at 10:30 PM: *"tPA infusing, wife by bedside."*

Then at 11:02 PM: *"Pt. remains with word salad speech and r sided weakness."*

It was months before I could tell my wife about the episode with tPA. I told her about touching my face and about the noise in my brain. She had wondered what I was doing. She saw me doing it and was listening to me talk "word salad," with *no* idea what I was thinking. We didn't get the complete story until after I received all the notes and reports from the hospital. The comments from the nurse noted what had been happening to me. My wife observed it too. I was *having* a stroke while *hearing* the popcorn popping as tPA dissolved my clot. There were few memories that day, but *that* was one of them. I have asked many nurses and doctors if they have ever heard about a patient who actually *heard* tPA working. They have never found anyone who had heard any noise. The doctors did say most patients were unconscious and therefore couldn't (consciously) hear it.

I was in the middle of a stroke when tPA stopped it cold. I would be quite a different person today if I had not received tPA. Of course, I didn't know the difference between tPA and aspirin. I was still conscious without being necessarily aware. I had no idea anything had happened until I felt the popcorn popping. I still didn't know what it was. The noise was so loud and so persistent it startled me. No one in the room heard what I had heard. It was all on the inside. Everyone in the room saw what I was doing. It felt like a toothache. When I attempted to explain what was happening to me, no real words came out. It was an important story *to me*. It was the beginning of understanding that something was happening. In many ways, it was the beginning of my recovery. I realized something was happening on the *inside*. It was the beginning of "seeing" my deficits. However, it would be quite a while before I could describe my experience to people on the *outside*.

The brain is an amazing device. I was not conscious of any memories other than a few spread over several days after my stroke. But I did *remember* those early memories, and I held on to them. As days, weeks, and months went by, everything I could remember was still linked to those few memories. Everything I know now has been traced back to my own "big bang."

At the very beginning, I could not explain to *myself* that I could not read, write, or speak well. After the first couple of days, I became more conscious of my thinking, and I was thinking about what was happening to me. That is still not to say I had any clear idea of my predicament. I was in a hospital and I knew it. I was in some kind of trouble and I knew that too. I could see other patients in the rooms around me who were physically worse than me. What I didn't know was: Why couldn't I go home? What was preventing me from going home? That was the problem. I couldn't say what I wanted to say.

But I could think. Eventually my thinking led me to discovering the deficits of each of my modalities. I didn't make a conscious decision about whether one modality was more or less impaired than another. Soon enough, I could tell *on the inside* that there was a ranking of each of the major deficits. The order of impairment for me was speaking, listening, reading, and writing. Speaking was the best and writing was the worst.

Once I got home, I started speaking with my wife, although that is not to say I did it frequently. My wife went to work, and I often slept until after she had left. When she came home, we had dinner, we talked about her day, and went for our normal walk. As we talked, I would often use "yes" and "no" answers. I was able to speak real words (as far as I knew). I used small words and simple words. I was still too confused (if I can say it that way) to attempt anything other than those that were easy. Using those "easy" words (which I thought *were* easy) turned out to be some of the more difficult problems from the start.

As I spoke, I could usually hear myself say simple words—using the *wrong* simple words. If I meant "yes," I often said "no." If I meant "she," I often said "he." If I meant "sister," I often said "brother." This goes on to this day. I was frustrated by the errors. That is not to say I was aware of all the errors. Frustration turned out to be a good thing. Frustration means you are aware of what is happening. Or at least aware enough to recognize the errors *in the moment* and recognize them earlier and earlier. This meant I might express what I *thought* was the right word, which turned out to be wrong. I would recant as soon as my mind noticed the wrong turn. The more I could recognize what was happening, the more I could assess and correct it.

The yes/no paradox was the tip of the aphasia iceberg. There were many examples of more complex ideas, often poorly composed. I didn't do it on purpose. My brain would fire off right messages that still went the wrong way. The brain is incredibly powerful, but each pathway can be damaged in different ways.

Mentally, I knew what I wanted to say. As soon as I started to say what I was thinking, a damaged pathway was taken. My thoughts moved at one speed and my expressed thoughts at another. As I have said, being aware is more than half the problem. The more complicated the expression, the more difficult it is to express. It goes back to the frustration that comes with aphasia. It is good to be aware of the deficits. They help us to get better by our talking. Given the frustration of being aware and *still* being unable to communicate properly, silence can still be golden. *Not* talking is so much easier than talking, given that you and the world around you must have the patience required to sort out the mess.

I had been speaking with my wife, family, and friends over the first couple of weeks since my stroke. I had not spoken in any formal or clinical way with anyone else. The doctors had said I needed to rest and let my brain "settle down." I didn't do much. I slept, ate, and watched TV. Three weeks after my stroke, I attended my first formal assessment with a speech-language pathologist, my speech therapist.

I remembered the assessment, but I *really* didn't understand it. I didn't *know* what I had said to the therapist until after I received the written report.

> *Verbal expression in conversation, with frequent phonemic and semantic paraphasias, as well as neologisms. For example, a pencil was called a "panger" and a whistle was called a "blesker." Pt.'s speech was also empty and without many content words, with pt. often referring to objects as "the thing" or "something" or "that."*

I read the report. At the time and for many months thereafter, I couldn't grasp what she had said. For one thing, I didn't know any of the clinical lingo of speech therapy. *Paraphasia* is a type of error with aphasia, and is described by unintended syllables, words, or phrases while speaking. It turned out that I did it quite a bit. *Neologisms* were new words or phrases that meant what I meant them to be, using these new words or nonsense words instead. Again, I wasn't aware of it at the time, and upon reading the report I still didn't remember I had said those unintelligible words. I must have done it, neologisms and all.

The "empty" words mentioned by the therapist were words I used regularly. I was looking for content words and when I couldn't find them, I used words like "things" or "that" as fillers until I could find the real words again. At the time, I used the filler words as the "easy" words. I didn't know I couldn't use anything else.

"Word-finding" activities became part of my practice *after* I became aware there were words in my brain that weren't lost. They were actually there and could be found. It took some amount of mental effort. The *effort* was tantamount to the experience-dependent neural plasticity that drives connectivity to occur.

It took a while for me to understand the headings, "verbal & written expressions," and "auditory & reading comprehensions" in the assessment. In my mind all I could think about was I had a problem, period. I had this new thing called "aphasia" and I was still a long way from understanding it. I had a sense that my speaking, listening, reading, and writing were all in trouble. I didn't get much further than that. Every time I read the assessment, I got confused. Maybe I wasn't confused as much as I was still having a hard time understanding the concept of the assessment. I understood all the words individually. Some of the words represented new and complex concepts that had been made more difficult for me to understand. I could "see" those words, but couldn't grasp their meaning. In the meantime, I read and reread my assessment and session reports, waiting for awareness to dawn.

My daughter arrived on the same day as my initial assessment, October 17, 2011. My next appointment with the therapist would not be for another week. We had nothing to do until then, so my daughter wanted me to practice. I didn't understand that the quizzes my daughter had created were almost identical to the "verbal expression" assessment conducted by my therapist. The prognosis is provided here.

> *Pt. was able to produce automatic sequences such as numbers 1–20, ABCs, days of the week and months with minimal cues; however, pt. was unable to produce these when presented out of order (i.e., count starting at the number 5 or say the days of the week starting at Tuesday).*

It was more than a little interesting that my daughter had encouraged me to start talking about numbers, letters, days of the week, months, etc., on the same day as my assessment. It had just been three weeks since my stroke. I had not been speaking much to anyone else. So I still had no real understanding about the issue of numbers, letters, and other items the therapists called, in her report, automatics.

After my daughter arrived, I practiced automatics on a regular basis. I recited the days of the week, months of the year, and the alphabet. I also rehearsed strings of numbers, 1-2-3-4-5-6-7-8-9-10, 10 to 20, and so on. As I repeated the automatics, I could tell I knew the words. I knew the days, the months, and the alphabet. I knew numbers. I could say them correctly, but only if they were in sequence. When my daughter asked for names, for example, of individual days of the week, I could not "say" the right word. I could see the word in my mind. I could find the right word and say it, but only if I started the string from the beginning. The right word arrived only if it was in the right position in the right sequence. For quite a while, I could not even say the right word without first whispering to myself the entire string, until I got to the word or number I needed and then saying it *out loud*.

I arrived at my first therapy session after a week of working with my daughter. My therapist provided me with a sheet of paper with what turned out to be the same sheet of paper my daughter had created the week before. The automatics contained numbers, days of the week, months of the year, and the alphabet. By then I was already proficient at saying all the words or numbers in a string. I had been saying them over and over for a week. What I still couldn't do was to be able to answer the question, "What day is tomorrow?" I knew the word. I knew what the word *tomorrow* meant in terms of the day. I still could not yet "compute" the answer such that I could find the words (or numbers) *other* than in sequence. I kept working with the word strings for several weeks. By the time I got to that point, I was now aware of the fact that my sequences were getting better. As time went by, I did less and less whispering. Whispering was subsumed into less *saying* and more *thinking* of what I was saying, before it was said.

Listening

When it came to listening, there were two different components of the same deficit. One was called listening (auditory) comprehension. Auditory comprehension describes a person's ability to understand the meaning of words he or she has heard. The other was called auditory processing. Auditory processing refers to how the brain "processes" sound. It must recognize and interpret those sounds with your language. At the time, I only understood the listening (auditory) comprehension portion of listening. The auditory processing portion didn't show up (meaning I didn't "see" it) until later, when it became a deficit. It was also called *rise time* or *slow rise time.*

Listening (Auditory) Comprehension

I had been listening to everyone around me. I talked with my therapists, my doctors, my family, my friends, and others. "Listening" didn't bother me. What I mean is, the *act of listening* didn't worry me. There was no overt effort on my part to hear what was said. I had even wondered if listening was not even a modality in the same tier as reading, writing, and speaking (like Pluto not being a planet). I never thought *listening* was somehow damaged. I could tell something didn't make sense. I wondered if I was not listening because I was thinking of something else. I certainly was not consciously aware of *not* understanding a word or a picture. The comprehension part of listening didn't occur to me. My first clue indicated I was having problems, given I was "guessing" at some of the answers. This is an excerpt from my assessment.

> *Listening (Auditory) Comprehension:*
> *Pt. was able to answer simple yes and no questions with 90% accuracy; however, complex yes and no questions were with only 50% accuracy and required frequent repetition and slow rate of speech. Pt. was able to follow 100% of single-step commands and only 40% of 2-step commands. Pt. able to answer 6/8 questions about a short paragraph correctly; however, pt. requested repetition and admitted to "guessing" on some.*

"Guessing" led me to understand I was not completely sure of my answers. I couldn't grasp what I once knew. I knew the logic of what an answer looked like. Even so, I couldn't understand the questions being asked of me. I felt there must have been a screen between the structure of a question asked and an answer given.

One simple question with only two answers (yes/no) was the beginning of thinking through a problem. As yes/no answers improved, I moved to more complex questions and multi-step instructions. I couldn't get them all right. I could understand sections of the multi-step question. However, I was unable to combine the individual (often right) sub-answers into a consolidated answer (often wrong). There was logic within the questions and answers. I could "see" them. Still, I could not "compute" the logic of the *many* into a completed *whole*.

It was like a puzzle. You find all the straight edges, the shapes, and then the colors. You arrange them appropriately and then look for similarities. Little by little, the puzzle is solved. It doesn't require intelligence as much as logic and an ability to look for patterns. That was how my brain solved this particular listening problem. The brain is a puzzle using logic, similarities, and patterns.

There was another aspect of working with a puzzle. You were looking for the orientation as well. Turning a piece one way or another provides a different perspective. You continued to try one piece and then another. It was always satisfying to find the piece you were looking for. *Not* finding it was satisfying in its own way too. There are only so many pieces that are *wrong* before you find the one that is *right*. Looking for the right piece is an exercise in futility, up to a point. After a bit, it becomes an exercise with a purpose. It then creates a mental "error condition" (a habit, if you like). I was becoming more aware of the habit of looking for the right answer. When it was a puzzle piece (or an answer) that fit, it felt good. The more I *felt*, the more aware I was of the contours of my deficits. The entire process of recovery is first measured by awareness. As I became more *aware* of errors, the more I could consciously *notice* the errors. And the more that were *noticed*, the more that were *corrected*.

Auditory Processing (Rise Time)

I had not been told anything about the "auditory processing" portion of the listening deficit. In my case, I was only aware of it by *experiencing* it. The deficit was part awareness and part attention. The more I experienced it in real time, the more I could recognize the deficit. It was called *rise time* or *slow rise time*. I found the information that described exactly what I had experienced. Rise time is related to an attention deficit within aphasia. It takes longer to shift from passive to active listening processing and, as a result, the first elements of a message are missed.

I was able to understand much of what I heard. Or what I should say was, I *thought* I could hear everything around me. But some things I couldn't "hear." There wasn't anything wrong with my ears. Only after many months did I understand there were other factors affecting my ability to listen, which didn't come from my ability to hear.

I had been talking with my wife and I realized as she talked, that I couldn't "hear" everything she was saying. That had gone on for quite a while before this realization hit me. I could hear what she was saying, but I couldn't "hear" for the first two or three words of her first sentence. I told my wife as soon as I recognized what was happening. It was a "eureka" moment. I told her I had been having a hard time understanding what she was saying—and it wasn't because I wasn't listening to her. As she talked, if I was not listening to her directly (or I was watching TV or listening to the radio), I "missed" the first two or three words. I'll admit, some amount of embarrassment came from that.

Someone with aphasia who has "lost" a lot in conversations might think it is always their fault. I could tell it wasn't mine.

I could tell the words I missed had been launched in my direction. I couldn't grasp them as they flew by, though. As a result, I couldn't "hear" them.

Once I had determined what had happened, there were several things I could do. Basically, there was too much "chatter" in the air. If I was watching TV, by the time my wife started to say something, I could not engage in time to hear it all. As soon as I heard a conversation was under way, I would break in and ask, "What was that?" I almost always say that now because I have already lost the first few words. Apparently, aphasia takes time to shift from one focused thought to another. As a result, the time it takes to "attend" the conversation is the time it takes to lose the first two to three words in the conversation.

If I was watching TV, or the phone was ringing, or another person in the room was conducting a conversation, there was too much noise. I could not separate one sound from another. When that happened, I would turn off the TV immediately so I could keep up with the conversation. Most healthy people don't have that kind of problem. Healthy people can listen to the radio, watch TV, and hear someone else talking, all at the same time. People with aphasia often think there is something wrong with them. I didn't think there was something wrong per se. After quite a while of not being able to *hear* what my wife was saying, I finally appreciated something was wrong. I could hear what I imagined was the reverberation of my wife's voice "getting through," until I could "hear" what she was saying. In the meantime, I had lost the first few words. I never knew I had that problem. I could never have *known* about the problem if I hadn't "listened hard" to what was going on around me. It was an "*ah-ha*" moment, for sure.

I came across an article called "The Role of Auditory Functions in Rehabilitation of Aphasic Individuals," by R. H. Brookshire. There was no date in the article; it appears to have been published in the 1970s. It was the first time I had heard of "rise time," with the exact explanation of my symptoms.

I also bought *Aphasia Rehabilitation* on March 12, 2012, in Waltham, MA. I didn't read the book until we moved to Florida. My notes in the book were dated November 28, 2012. While sitting on my couch in St. Augustine, Florida, I read about rise time for the first time in a book about aphasia.

> *Rise Time. The patient whose processing system is characterized by slow rise time tends to miss the initial portions of incoming auditory messages because his/her processing system takes a greater amount of time to shift from a passive nonprocessing state to an active processing state. Therefore, development and selection of treatment tasks were selected with this factor in mind.* (Ross and Spencer)

Rise time is a big problem, with social implications. The symptoms of rise time make it sound like you *can't* hear, you don't *want* to pay attention, or you are too *frustrated* to listen. It could be all of those things. Without being informed about that particular deficit, you might never know.

Apparently, it is a categorical (real) deficit, but low in the totem pole of speech therapy. In any case, rise time is something a therapist should talk about with one's patients. Otherwise, neither the patient nor the caregiver will know anything about it. It will be invisible to the family and friends, and be framed by the social difficulties that gave rise to rise time.

Reading

Reading proved to be a confusing time. I couldn't read, yet it wasn't the same as saying a few words as if I *could* read. That's why I call it confusing. I couldn't explain the deficits of reading even though I knew the words that went into the sentences I was unable to say.

After my stroke I assumed I could read. It was still too soon for me to fully grasp what was not yet in view. I could see real words. Days of the week, months of the year, and numbers were all words I could recognize. I could understand each of the words. I could read those words (in my mind). As a result, I thought I *could* read and was *able* to read. I didn't know that *some* of the factors of reading were individually damaged. I could read individual words, but could not read a sentence with meaning. My grammar and syntax were gone. The links between the rules and the meaning of words had to be reconnected. I wouldn't know it for a while that my reading deficit included working memory problems as well (Caspari).

For weeks after my stroke but before my therapy, I didn't do anything. I didn't read. I didn't write. I certainly didn't speak much. That is not to say I *knew* I had these problems. I existed without any real comprehension of my life at the time.

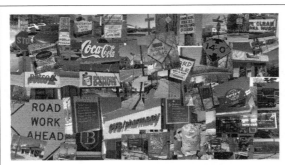

3-1 Street signs in Waltham and Watertown, MA.

I did walk. I walked for miles. I could read (most) signs on the street:

street signs, traffic signs, directional signs, historical signs, warning signs, hospital signs, airport signs, and police signs (figure 3-1).

I could read signs at all kinds of stores. I could read signs at food stores, coffee shops, restaurants, gas stations, movies, pharmacies, pet stores, post office, libraries, universities, churches, florists, banks, dentists, and doctors. Again, I could read the signs and interpret most of what I was seeing. There were usually only one or two words on a sign. I knew what they were and what they did.

I could read menus from restaurants. I had been having breakfast with a friend for years. After my stroke, we continued. Most of the menus provided information about the meal, plus pictures with eggs, ham, bacon, pancakes, and coffee for breakfast, and other meals for lunch or dinner. If I couldn't say what I wanted to say, I could point at the pictures. The server would also point at the item and confirm what I meant, and then I could indicate yes or no.

As I read signs every day, I was beginning to understand I was conscious of being able to read those words. As the signs got more complex, I came up against (what had to have been) the mental pressure (anxiety, worry, concern) of not being able to understand what was in front of me.

I continued reading signs, joined by new activities with my speech therapist. It seemed I was progressing quickly, like a newborn baby that went from babbling to letters to words to reading. I progressed from being unable to read, write, or speak well, to being able to do those things within eleven months.

As weeks went by, I could study the activities provided by my therapist. I could read the "pictured" words of glasses, pants, guitar, suitcase, refrigerator, box, camera, bell, and candle on a page. I could read the fill-in-the-blank activities, including pen and … ink, needle and … thread, pots and … pans, and bow and … arrow.

I could read "Feature Comparisons" activities provided by my therapist with Yes or No answers. I answered the question, "Is chicken broth thinner than clam chowder?" correctly. I got 8 out of 10 right that day.

With so much information to digest, you would have thought I really *could* read. What I didn't know at the time was the difference between reading a word or two (and their images) versus being able to read more complex information with meaning. That is where it broke down. It was easy for me to understand simple words and signs. The more complicated the concepts, the more difficult it was for me to interpret the reading.

One Feature Comparisons activity I got wrong was, "Does a plain have more trees than a forest?" It was a relatively simple concept that was still too involved for me to grasp. A Yes/No question is one thing. A "compare and contrast" question, while easy before my stroke, became part of the deficits. I recognized my mental thesaurus was damaged too.

Given that I could see all kinds of words around me, I realized my reading deficit had something to do with the rules and grammar of the language and not so much the words per se. Many words contained meaning within the structure of the words. I knew what they meant. As I tried to connect words to make a sentence, it didn't happen. I could only read one word at a time.

It appeared that those words were hidden behind a closed curtain. As I opened the curtain, I could read the word. In order to read the *next* word, I had to close the first curtain before I could open the next. After reading the second word, I could no longer remember the first. I could do that for each word. I would remember the word in front of me. I could not remember the word I had just seen. It was a one-word-at-a-time view. Like the big binoculars at the Empire State Building. You get a quarter's worth of the view. Then it closes; it's a blank. I experienced a long string of words in a sentence one quarter at a time. I could no longer integrate the collective meaning of words I once knew. In some ways it was a memory issue as well. I couldn't remember enough of the meaning of each of the words in the string to make an intelligent rendering of the sentences.

I used Google and Wikipedia, an online encyclopedia, to gather more information about my stroke and aphasia. I called them Wiki Notes. I printed out each article or online note and read them. I highlighted the new and interesting parts and used them to look for new information. *Stroke* led to *ischemia* led to *tPA* led to *clotting*. *Speech pathology* led to *semantic memory* led to *neurons* led to *aphasia* led to *Broca's area*.

Every day led me to new information about my brain and what was wrong with it. Of course, not unlike the signs I was reading on the street, the shorter the title, the easier to understand. As I read the articles I added margin notes in addition to the highlighting. As I read articles that still did not make sense to me, one-word notes helped me distill what I was thinking. Not all of those notes make sense, even today, without the context of the article. Words like "noticeable, masked, perception of change, left back, dendrites, neuron, brain, and cerebullum [*sic*]" were among them. Not unlike the shorter signs, I could only write one or two words before getting into a problem trying to write longer sentences.

Some ideas from Wiki Notes led me to buy some books. However, it is not the same as *reading* those books. I bought the books because of their title and the table of contents. I couldn't read the rest of the book. I figured I would be able to read them at some point. I wanted to be ready when I needed them.

The first book was *Synaptic Self: How Our Brains Become Who We Are* (LeDoux). I have read the book several times since then. I now understand much better how the brain coordinates thoughts (feelings, attitudes, ideas) through interconnected synapses.

For a while, I wasn't terribly good at reading Wiki Notes. The more I read, though, the more my reading improved. I printed the Wiki Notes about *Synaptic Self.* There was a margin note I had written: *"Bought start ~~word~~ book notes."* Not bad for a short sentence with no grammar. There were index card notes in the book with my handwriting. I must have been reading the book. I must have been learning *something.* There must have been a huge difference between what I was *thinking* versus what I was trying to write *about* what I was thinking. Of course I didn't know what it meant at the time (or even today.) I was practicing my language and that was all that mattered. Here is the note.

> *Other decision between us and there all is the stroke always ~~es~~ us be 'hear' about it (so tangible) all but all of us in owe the brain. Another the symtoms [sic] (of stroke) I no not have seem any significant symtoms [sic] in any way being ~~bout~~ there of brain.* (Index card)

Another entry on an index card was labeled "page 133," with the page titled "Remembering Who We Are." This entry used real words that still make no sense. Practice provided the feedback required to notice what was wrong and correct it.

> *Memoring [sic] facts but are stories in past but stories in facts in past be didn't below story into now storied absent the past.* (Index card)

I got better at reading without necessarily being conscious of improvement on a day-to-day basis. I read regularly, but was still unaware of the influence of the institution called "practice."

At the time I was not aware that my reading and writing were equally "bad." Only later I became aware of the difference between "good" and "bad." I saved all the evidence and that was important. There would *not* have *been* a comparison, *without* a "good" and a "bad." Practice made it happen.

There was one more thing about the difference between my past performance and my improvement over time. I developed a spreadsheet to collect my Wiki Notes and the books I had bought. Each item included a short title, several notes, and the date when it was printed or purchased.

Going from "bad" to "good," I would not have known my improved condition without the time scale. I printed my Wiki Notes and threw them into several boxes, where they stayed until we moved to Florida. It was only then I saw there was a date on every printed page. Every book had an invoice with the date of the order. Once I entered the records, I could start to see the difference between a *now* and a *then*. I had been thinking *then* (and had tried to express my intentions using fractured grammar) versus *now*, with a healing (not quite whole) grammar.

As the story progresses, I went from losing my grammar to getting it back again. As far as I could tell, no one had ever told me "my grammar was gone." Eventually I was aware of some of my deficits—although I didn't realize I had "lost my grammar" until later. Individual problems littered throughout my therapy reports certainly inferred that something along that line had happened.

I got the reports each week. There was no overarching context about the depth and detail of each of the modalities and the integrated nature of the deficits. The context of recovery appeared bit by bit. My weekly reports indicated increases in my performance. Increasing to 80% accuracy of "sentence completions" and 90% of "phrase completions" was not the same as the *organic* feedback provided *by* me and *to* me. I didn't know it at the time. I was not aware of any mental "sessions" sending me "reports" week by week. Each modality provided some amount of intensive (and neural) feedback that allowed recovery to occur.

I have always loved the movie, *L.A. Story*. Steve Martin talked to an electronic sign on the freeway. The sign displayed messages in the form of metaphors, riddles, and cryptic advice about love and life. The messages were just for him.

I read signs everywhere I saw them. It was easy. They were short. Since I didn't talk to many humans, the signs were almost as good. I talked to the signs, reading aloud, as I walked. Initially there were easy signs: STOP, YIELD, CAUTION. Then I moved on to more difficult signs, ROAD WORK AHEAD, PERMIT PARKING ONLY, SALE PENDING. Traffic signs progressed to street signs, to school signs, and then church signs.

There were many churches in my town, and the church signs got longer. They had prayers and sentiments, events with announcements, and electric signs with important information. They also had memorial plaques commemorating history, battles, and the community. There was one church I saw almost every day. Believe it or not, I could not pronounce several (very easy) words from a particular plaque. So, every day I would talk to the sign (it wouldn't listen). I stood right in front of it and therefore, right in front of the church, with a clear view from the street (figure 3-2).

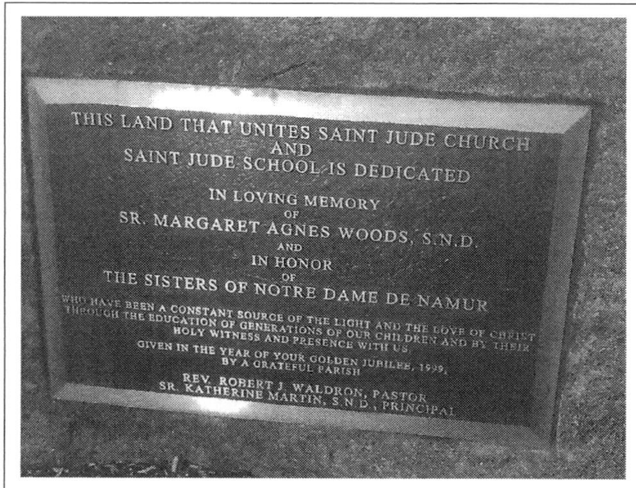

3-2 Picture of the "LAND THAT UNITES" Church plaque, Tuesday, November 22, 2011.

Every day before I started talking, I checked around. There was a police station across the street and lots of police cars. I wondered if they were wondering about me. The more I talked to my sign, the more likely someone else must have seen (and must have been concerned about) me … talking out loud to a church sign across from a police station. It was probably not the best therapy I could pick. That's why I used pictures instead of talking to myself!

The sign at the church included the words "Land" and "Unites." I used those words in my diary as well. I was trying to figure out how to pronounce these very simple words. Eventually I "found" how to say "Land." I realized I *could* say the word "Sand." I transposed an *S* to an *L* and I had found it. La-La-La-Land. I was excited about those two words. I couldn't pronounce the word "Unites" for a long time. I kept on saying the word, "Units" most of the time. The day finally came when I could say, "THIS LAND THAT UNITES…." It was a good sign.

Writing

The first time I wrote anything after my stroke was during my home-schooled therapy. As mentioned previously, my daughter came for two weeks to help me. She was a neuroscience grad in college and knew a little bit about aphasia. She created some written exercises including days of the week, months of the year, the alphabet, numbers, and time. She knew enough to know I was having problems with each of these issues. I had been having a hard time saying the easiest things. I used the home-schooled exercises every day. I stumbled over the words (letters and numbers) and realized I was stumbling in different ways.

Therapists call it automatics. I could spell most of the words, so that wasn't the problem. The problem was I could not "find" the items spontaneously. If I initiated word sets from the beginning (Monday, January, 1, or *A*), I could recite the entire set, hence automatics. If I was asked to respond to a word in the middle of the set (Thursday, June, 13, or *M*), I could not do it. I said Tuesday instead of Thursday, or July instead of June. I could find the right word eventually, but only by reciting the entire set. When I arrived at the right word, I repeated it over and over, hoping it would help. I could not *assign* the right word to the slot I wanted to say, spontaneously. It was an important realization. The sequence was defective, not the words themselves. I kept repeating the sets as quickly as I could. They felt like they were getting easier, or stronger.

As I tried writing the automatics, it still took longer to "find" them and write them (if at all), rather than speaking them out loud. So I continued to recite the sequences to "get to" the word. Then I wrote it down.

After a couple of weeks, I was getting better. It wasn't perfect. By then I didn't even *try* to find the out-of-sequence word. I would go as fast as I could to get to the right word (often to myself). Then I could *say* or *write* the right word, *as if* I didn't have the original problem. The manual process slowly disappeared as the automatic sequence took over.

There are still times when I can't "find" the right words. If I was in a noisy place, there have been times when I missed a beat. If I was speaking to a crowd, I would explain to the group I *had* missed a beat. I also asked if *they* had seen it happen too. That was always fun. The automatics deficits were a good example of how cell networks "exercise" to rebuild what has been damaged. Practice, repeat, and repeat again.

After a week of home-schooled therapy, my formal aphasia therapy got under way. My therapist had noted in her report that I had been practicing with automatics for a week with my daughter. She reiterated the out-of-order problem and provided written exercises to work on at home. The rest of the session explained the basics of the alphabet, numbers, and words.

Later that week, I started using my diary. I had found some black-and-white composition books and figured I should use them. I had used them like diaries or journals before. I actually started my diary by copying the exercises from my therapist. The first paragraph was freestyle, with almost perfect spelling and imperfect grammar. There were several pages of well-done copied lists of animals, food, states, and body parts. In between the lists was other similar freestyle writing. None of it made any sense. I could tell there was a difference in the way it looked to me. Freestyle writing from a person with aphasia appears like it took more effort. When I copied lists provided by my therapist it felt "easy," less effort. It was hard to understand. It felt like the difference between hard or smooth, jagged or linear, and between "working hard" to produce my words versus the lists generated by someone else. It *felt* like that to me even if I couldn't express it. This was the first entry in my diary.

> *Design being ~~calenent~~ calendar and and day of the design. Day is ~~deig~~ during "day" and "month". (Brain settle set one age of set settle). Lessons ~~B~~ due spelling and sending of dual spelling (10/27/2011).*

As we read this *now*, what I said back *then* didn't make any sense. It made sense to me at the time. I wrote, read, and reread the entries so many times and they always looked "fine" to me. They kept looking "fine" until I had crossed the threshold of awareness. But I am getting ahead of myself. That paragraph looked as "fine" as the written lists (that *were* fine) which I had added to my diary. In addition, my initial therapy included writing fill-in-the-blank exercises (with pictures of the items) from my therapist. I wrote: brush, screwdriver, baseball, ruler, key, knife, mirror, lamp, hammer, toothbrush, cup, coin, sock, and dice. I got most of them right. Some were misspelled (which I corrected). It was an interesting thing. At the instant of writing something wrong, I was *aware* it was wrong and corrected it. Awareness continued to be a key to recovery.

It seemed *time* was the issue behind awareness. I was beginning to tell some of the circuits were slow. When I was healthy, I could read, write, and speak simultaneously. I didn't think about time as an entity, like food or fuel. Time was just *there*. Once I had my stroke, I could tell there was an appreciable delay between what I wanted to say (in my mind) and the time lag it took to announce the word in my mouth.

Illumination was a sheet of lightning (in my mind), without any realization there were individual strokes of lightning, each with their own beginning, middle, and end. As I slowed down (because of my stroke), I could see the individual strokes. So, when a bolt went haywire, I could see it (in real time) and still have the time to redirect or send another message quickly. In any case, what I thought was instantaneous only seemed that way. I could now see at least four to five appreciable messages I could discern in a second. I assumed an instantaneous message took 200 milliseconds or *less*. I practiced saying four or five short words in a second. If I was healthy, every one of those words would be right.

I realized that if I made a mistake, it didn't take a lot of time to notice an error. I figured that being slow meant it took twice as long and that meant it took 400 ms *rather* than 200 ms. That was still pretty fast. Slow enough for me to observe errors in the making, yet fast enough to realize it as wrong and still have time to launch another missile under 1,000 ms. Some deficits did take longer. Some deficits had been taken "off line," such that they had to wait to be recharged completely.

While completing the fill-in-the-blank exercises, I had also been writing in my diary on the same day. Similarly, I had misspelled other words in my diary. At the moment of writing what was wrong, I was *also* aware of the errors and fixed them. Interestingly, there was only one word that still didn't make sense ("mouche.") I was *aware* it was wrong (and added a [sp?]) to alert me it was *not* a real word. I couldn't figure out what I meant. Misspelling words was one kind of problem and grammar another. Here is an example.

> *Bring the day? Bring sometime say in exacting yesterday the timely in different if anything tabling. 'My brain in you the spelling' my thing thought mind-spelling thing we are spelling there misspell in mouche (sp?) [sic]. Great I lots lots I must all (10/31/2011).*

So, on the same day, there were two different deficits with similar characteristics utilizing two different modalities. The fill-in-the-blank exercises were easy. Most of my answers were right. Yet later that day I wrote entire sentences that were wrong. What I didn't realize (and never did until 11 months later) was that the grammar in my diary induced its own kind of deficit. As I read (and reread) my diary, everything continued to look fine (to me). The words were spelled correctly. The problem was the arrangement of the words that didn't make any sense. I was aware I could spell. For the most part, the words were right. If a word was misspelled, I could usually "tell" it was wrong, and had "time" to fix it. However, when it came to grammar, I was unaware that the rules themselves were wrong. I couldn't "think my way" through it like I did with spelling. The underlying foundation of the grammar problem was unawareness of the deficit itself.

Part 2

Beyond Speech Therapy

PART 2 INTRODUCTION

My therapy was like all speech therapy: word-finding exercises and repetition. My "language problems" were all I knew. Aphasia was a new word I had never heard before my stroke. Word-finding exercises and repetition were the sum total of my therapy. I had been told I was having problems with my language and, in particular, being unable to find certain words. That was true. I could tell I couldn't say some words. It bothered me. I actually could *see* those words in my mind. I couldn't conjure the right words even though they were on the tip of my tongue. The "tip of my tongue" words were close yet far away at the same time. I could *see* it but couldn't *say* it. The depths of my language problems were just below the surface. I didn't know what it would take to fix it. It was a bad problem, but how bad could it be?

I attended my therapy sessions with lots of questions and my questions weren't always the best. For one, I couldn't explain what I wanted to ask. The therapist used the right words with her responses. I couldn't put it all together. We tried to communicate. On my part, there was a mismatch between what was said and what was heard. I couldn't "remember" what I had said *to* the therapist. I couldn't "hear" what I had heard *from* the therapist. If presented individually, I could hear the individual words. In the moment, I couldn't remember (or remember them long enough) to gather the meaning the words possessed. As a result, the gaps made it difficult to communicate. But I could *think*. Thinking was the first tool I needed. I didn't *consciously* devise a plan. It seemed to assemble itself.

Speech therapy and word-finding exercises were a small part of a much larger plan of recovery. The word-finding exercises were appealing. But after the exercises, there was no time left to explore my problems with my therapist, before the next patient arrived. I had to invent my accidental therapy far beyond speech therapy. I understood there was an environment that would provide more enrichment than speech therapy alone.

It seemed a natural sequence was leading me towards enrichment. Somewhere in my brain, I must have known I would get better. I wasn't consciously aware of it at the time. The more I *thought* about the problems, the more activities appeared. I didn't make a conscious decision to act one way or another. I didn't *decide* to think. Thinking is what thinking does. The more I *thought* provided more of the *substance* of what I was thinking, like grinding grain into flour.

I started walking and it wasn't such a big deal. Thinking shadowed me at every step. What came first, the chicken or the egg? As I started to think more about my problems, I recorded my thoughts. I didn't know why. I understood I had some problems. Some of those problems were invisible for me to appreciate. The physical evidence of what was wrong would help me understand how to make it right. I collected the evidence long before I was able to analyze it.

Once I had accumulated a critical mass of data for my diary, voice memos, and pictures, I appreciated different perspectives of the same (thought) events. There were indications in my diary, voice memos, and pictures of the same thoughts that had appeared on the same day. Each modality provided its own version of the same message with the same feedback. Each altered version contributed to a more complete whole.

Speech therapy helped. Nevertheless, many more therapeutic activities were needed to advance the process of recovery. Speech therapy is a small fraction of the therapeutic energy available. Each of those activities ran in parallel with speech therapy.

My recovery didn't happen *because* of my speech therapy. It didn't happen *instead* of my speech therapy. It didn't happen *in spite of* my speech therapy. My recovery happened as a *result* of my speech therapy *plus* new therapeutic activities *embedded* in an enriched environment.

No one had explained this to me. I am not a speech therapist or a neuroscientist. I am a stroke survivor. My recovery was ameliorated in light of the novel therapeutic activities that contributed to it. And there wasn't a single element, or two, out of the many that accounted for the improvement. Every activity was woven into the same engineered fabric. The interaction of each of the elements contributed to the strength of all. It would be impossible to recognize the active ingredients of one or two elements as the only *real* reason for improvement.

Researchers have been trying to determine if certain ingredients are *more* important, *more* essential, and *more* necessary. In the course of their studies, it appeared that all the ingredients are poured into a mold of an enriched environment which protects, defends, and heals the brain when *all* of them are present. To do otherwise would jeopardize the enriched environment that provides plasticity and the ability to change.

CHAPTER FOUR

WALKING IS THINKING

Methinks that the moment my legs begin to move, my thoughts begin to flow ....

—Henry David Thoreau

Solvitur ambulando – It is solved by walking.
—Diogenes the Cynic, 4th-century BC Greek philosopher

When you have a stroke, it takes a while before you can do anything. You are groggy and can barely tell what day it is. For the first couple of weeks, I couldn't eat or sleep well, or read or write. I couldn't think in any organized way. It is the definition of having a stroke. I was told to be careful about walking (or driving) until I was sure I knew my way around. (Look out for Silver Alert notifications!) When I had walked around the floor at the hospital, I was worried I might get lost.

So I didn't walk without my wife. I didn't leave on my own until after my wife was sure I knew my way home. According to my calendar, I started walking on Tuesday, October 11, 2011. I walked for 12 miles that day. The calendar indicated another 12 miles on the next day, so I must have made it home!

Walking *was* thinking for me. Walking takes time. The longer I walked, the more thinking presented itself. If I was walking about 3 miles/hour, a typical walk would take 4 hours or so. So there was lots of time to consider (reflect, contemplate, ruminate) my situation. Why not? It was a beautiful day. Exercise is good. Plus I brought money in case I needed to eat (and I always like to eat). There was nothing to do *but* think. As I walked, I spent hours thinking about my problems. Not that I knew what those problems were at the time. I had yet to meet with my therapist. The assessment was a week away and my first speech therapy session was a week after that. Unable to express my thoughts, I walked and waited.

As I walked, signs were all around me. I knew there was something wrong with my language. As I looked at the signs, I could see (observe, recognize, notice) the words, and *thought* (imagined, perceived, knew) I could read the signs. What I mean was, I "got the impression" I could read them. I could read all kinds of different signs. I read stop signs, traffic signs, warnings signs, and many others. Some words I could *not* read. Some signs I couldn't even pronounce. "Brandeis" and "Bentley" were among those that appeared only in my mind. I couldn't say them out loud. The words were corrupted in such a way that I couldn't jump from a mental appreciation for the words (that I could *see*) into a physical set of syllables (that I couldn't *say*).

I took one of several different walking routes, depending on the day and the weather. The Bentley route took me through the Bentley College campus several days a week. I would look at every "Bentley" sign, hoping to find a hint as to how to say it. I was aware I couldn't pronounce it *in my mind*. I looked at the word. I looked at each letter. I practiced trying to say

Bentley, including using the syllables *Bent* and *ley*. It still didn't make any sense to me at the time. But I was becoming aware—a good thing.

From my perspective (which is to say, *in my mind*), there was an observer observing my thoughts. I could tell there was a "third person" talking to a "first person" and I was both of those people. Somehow, the act of walking allowed "me" to parse my thoughts into both the thoughts *thought* and the thoughts *observed*. Then I realized there were probably more than two. I realized *I* was observing the observer watching my thoughts. I thought about this and concluded this wasn't a "split personality" type of problem. I didn't think it was a mental problem. It seemed natural to watch the world around me through the eyes of another observer. I realized that many people have the capacity to study and observe their own thoughts. Otherwise called *metacognition*, I was monitoring my own thought processes. Aphasia presented me with the opportunity.

My stroke permitted one part of me to observe my deficits while another part of me was working just fine. I spent hundreds of hours walking and thinking about my deficits. Without any physical evidence, the only tool I had was thinking. The observer had the capacity to study without anything to work with. As I walked, I talked for a month until I started recording my voice. At that point I had discovered another tool. Voice recording provided the physical evidence of my thinking.

Walking *was* thinking. It was a Möbius strip. A Möbius strip is created by taking a paper strip and giving it a half-twist, and then joining the ends of the strip together to form a loop. If an ant were to crawl along the length of this strip, it would return to its starting point, having traveled the entire length of the strip (on both sides of the original paper) without ever crossing an edge. In this case, walking was on one side and thinking on the other. What I didn't know was that walking would provide the fodder for thinking. That is the way a Möbius strip works.

No one told me to walk. No one told me to think, either. Reconstructing the concept of aphasia recovery started with walking. People with aphasia (especially at the beginning) are largely unaware of their deficits. They are unaware of the concept of recovery. They are unaware of *being* unaware of any number of conscious and unconscious activities that can convey recovery.

Walking facilitated thinking. If it is your habit to walk, great. If you have been consciously motivated about your recovery, that is great too. If you have not been *consciously* motivated to practice your language or think about your deficits, then there is another path. Walking is the way.

Formal therapy provided some assistance, but not enough. Short classes with limited sessions do not provide the therapeutic energy needed to drive the ever-more-active recovery. An unconscious fuse can still be lit to a conscious appreciation of recovery-in-the-making.

When it comes to therapy, many stroke survivors do what they are told, or less. Much of what they are told to do are tasks and exercises with an objective of improved language. No one will tell them to think. No one would ever do that. Yet the proximate step for thinking is walking. It is something a clinician *can* do. A patient who is still too unaware at several different levels might be unmotivated, uninterested, or uncooperative to deal with the tasks. Despite this, walking and thinking can provide the patient any number of benefits.

A recent study described the various modes of neural processing. One is called the *default mode*, which allows the mind to wander. The default mode permits the mind to engage in internally focused thought. It includes "effortful abstract thinking, especially with socioemotional relevance." (Immordino-Yang) Walking lets the mind wander and reflect on personal memories, visualizing the future, and internally focusing mental processing. The researchers use the term *constructive internal reflection*. Walking provides the capacity to reflect on emerging awareness and deficits.

Walking offers immediate stimulation from something other than word exercises and watching TV. Experiencing, or engaging your sensations, provides the active ingredients of thinking. Walking improves health. Your heart beats faster, using more oxygen to build muscles as well as the brain. Walking provides new connections for brain cells, which enhances memory and retention. Walking is another step towards recovery. Walking is effortless for many aphasia patients. For those who are still unaware of their deficits, walking can provide a secret elixir to thinking and recovery. I walked *in order* to think. Therapists can't tell patients to think, but they can instruct patients to walk.

CHAPTER FIVE

PROBLEM SOLVING IS LEARNING

The path of least resistance and least trouble is a mental rut already made. It requires troublesome work to undertake the alteration of old beliefs.

—John Dewey

As I walked around town, I thought about what had really happened to my brain. I didn't have a lot to go on. I had never thought about my mind before and how it (actually) worked. So I started an inventory of what I *did* know. I knew I had a stroke. I knew some part of my brain had been damaged. I knew I had lost some cells from the loss of oxygen. I had some sense that my language was damaged. I couldn't pin it down. I couldn't tell if one aspect of my language or another was demonstrably wrong. It felt bad (odd, different, strange).

I walked for miles, reflecting (thinking, wondering, musing, pondering) about the sensation of losing *something* without being able to describe the loss. I thought about the loss of cells from the stroke. I thought about the connection between the lost cells and my damaged language. The inventory was meager, but trace evidence was a start.

What does it mean to be *thinking hard* about something? For most people, *thinking hard* typically means trying hard to find an answer. It represents a mental effort to solve a problem. It is usually accompanied by a physical expression, eyes closed, a grimace, or stroking the chin. Sound familiar? I had no idea that the act of *thinking hard* (problem solving, by any other name) would actually bring about more clarity. Every act of *thinking hard* provides a necessary and sufficient change in the brain that underlies learning.

Lost Cells versus Lost Words?

I actually conjured up the problem of the lost cells. I had always been good with math. So I thought in math terms. I had been told I had lost about 2 billion cells from my stroke. I imagined that my lost cells must have taken whole words with them. Given the 2% number of the 100 billion neurons, I assumed I had lost 2% of my vocabulary.

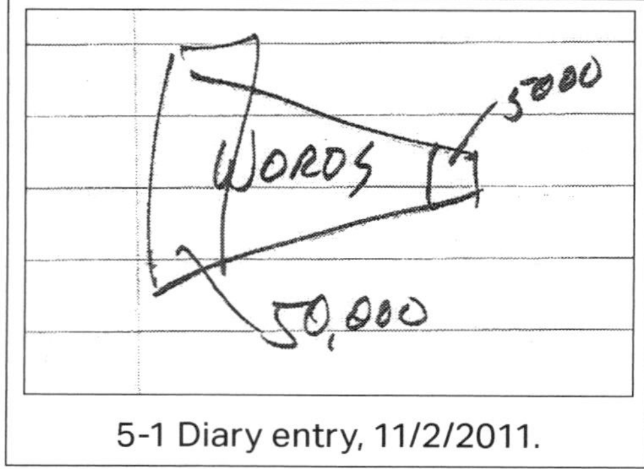

5-1 Diary entry, 11/2/2011.

There are about 50,000 words in the vocabulary of an adult. I drew a picture (figure 5-1) that looked a lot like a traffic cone on its side. I drew the word "Words" on it. On the base of the funnel, I wrote "50,000." I wrote "5,000" as the number of lost words. I had no reason for the discrepancy except to blame it on my stroke! As a result I made a guess that a large number, or amount, of my vocabulary was lost, based on the lost cells.

I had never known how the brain and memory actually (physically) operate. I had never known how a stroke worked either. My engineer brain simply looked at things proportionately and came up with the number. Lost cells = Lost words was the equation, but it wasn't the answer.

Within days I started thinking differently. There was something wrong. I was beginning to see various degrees of errors across every domain. As I was working with my day-to-day exercises, I could tell that many words were impaired in one way or another, but none were "lost." (There were some words I couldn't "see," but that wasn't because they were "lost." It was a different issue and a different deficit.)

Within days, I made a new decision. The Lost cells = Lost words did *not* work. My original thought about losing words was wrong. I realized that individual, discrete words were *not* contained in folders or files. I thought the files in the brain were organized similarly to a computer. It wasn't the case. I could tell many words were bent or scratched in one way or another. Yet, no words were lost forever.

I walked for miles before I started my diary. I must have been thinking about it for a while. Soon after starting my diary, I drew the "Lost cells = Lost words" equation. If I had not kept my diary, I would not have known what I was thinking. More importantly, I would not have had the *evidence* of what I was thinking. I probably forgot and remembered it more than once, until I wrote it down in my diary. The evidence was what I needed. Otherwise it was just a dream.

Parts of Parts

Once I knew that words were not kept in a file, I looked for a new explanation. In an earlier note, I had reviewed my pronunciation of the alphabet. At the time, 13 letters were OK. The other 13 letters weren't necessarily completely wrong. They weren't right, either. There was something wrong about each one. I wrote a full page about "pronunciation," using "slur, articulation, out loud, worthiness, and a different wrong."

My personal theory of "parts of parts" came from my work in shipbuilding. We built "parts" and "pieces" (built by smaller parts) that were generic. Many parts could be oriented one way or another into any number of different pieces. Many pieces could also be arranged to become many different items. It was a great analogy. The evidence made a lot of sense even though my language still couldn't.

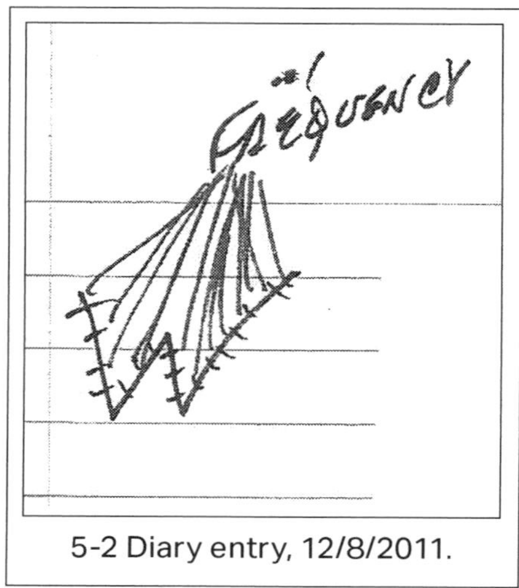

5-2 Diary entry, 12/8/2011.

It seems when I mispronounced a word, the letter was the culprit. The letters themselves were not all right or all wrong. There seemed to be some mechanism that contributed smaller parts to bigger parts to letters. It felt like some of the smaller parts were damaged. Depending on the critical mass of the damage to the smaller parts, the assembled bigger parts could also have been damaged, as well as a letter and even a word.

I drew a big picture of the letter *W* (figure 5-2). I put slashes on each line of the letter, indicating a number of short lines all joined to become the letter. I thought individual "letters" weren't put into files either. I was sure the letters (and everything else brain-language-wise) were identified down into what I had imagined were cells. I figured the cells were something generic. The cell networks (for letter- and word-type entities) must have been rolled up to become units "used" as something perceptual. Of course, I didn't know any of this at the time. I was using metaphorical drawings to explain what I otherwise didn't know. It was like recounting a dream. Get it quick, before it disappears.

I imagined that combinations of those cells were networked to form one letter or another. I am sure there had to have been a number of "cell-letter networks" with the same letter such that they formed a large number of populations (of cell-letter networks). Think of it as "alphabet soup." In that bowl, hundreds (if not thousands) of every letter (or every cell-letter network) were floating there. When words or sentences were formed they used letters consisting of networked, cell-letter networks. They were then dredged up from the pot to join whatever larger entities were needed. With aphasia, there is "*No soup for you*!" (Quote credit: *Seinfeld* TV Series, "The Soup Nazi," 1995)

At that point, I had begun to assume (in my brain, anyway) my language was being built up from cells to networks, and from networks to critical masses of network entities. I thought the damage had come the same way. Lost neurons affected networks and lost networks affected critical masses of networks and so on. This text accompanied the *W* drawing:

What alphapet [*sic*] *or words setting out in the brain a seeing "parts" of the words the last parts not notwithstanding of an whole part, parts and words. I became "blown up" in our an brain & tell are up up behariour* [*sic*] *outside while needed.* (Diary, 12/8/2011)

The billions of cells lost were (probably) selected at random. As a result I didn't lose a preponderance of one letter or one word. The lost cells essentially took some "off the top" of a random set of neuron networks.

Some networks were probably disbanded as a result of falling below some required "critical mass" for acquiring letters and words. It seemed falling below the critical mass still didn't mean it was "gone" as much as it was faded. I tried to say things (and sometimes came close) that had a "fading" quality to them. I would need to recruit additional networks to speak perfectly again. "Recruiting" of additional cells and cell networks was the textbook definition of "practice." I needed to practice by building up parts of parts, pieces, and networks to make my language work again.

It appeared that the brain was in possession of *knowing* what had happened with my stroke. It seemed the mind *knew* it was going to have to reassemble (and grow) a number of cells and networks to improve. It seemed to know half the battle would be done by *thinking* about the problems. Conscious (and sometimes unconscious) *thinking* stimulated active *doing*. The experience of *doing* was converted into the physical process of growing new "parts" of neurons (dendrites, synapses) which can supplement the function of the lost cells.

Think of it like exercising any muscles. Other muscle groups are called on to do what the body wants them to do. Those muscle groups are distinct entities, like the arms, legs, shoulders, and hands. A message sent from the brain responds with increased glucose, oxygen, and sweat. As a result, those muscles get bigger.

The same "growing" function happens with the brain. Solving mental problems is, in its own way, equivalent to running a mile or lifting weights. It is like building *mental* muscles. Damaged writing, reading, or speaking can only be improved through practice. Practice initiated the growing function to occur. The more the practice, the more the function grows. Resolving the deficits of aphasia is a test of mental effort with a physical twin. You can't have one without the other. My brain got better with mental sweat and tears.

One Syntax Or Two?

I had been thinking about the difference between my ability to speak versus my ability to write. Just outlining the problem was an important step because it was framed by my deficits. I didn't know the exact conditions of each of my spoken and written deficits. I was only aware of one modality being so much worse than the other.

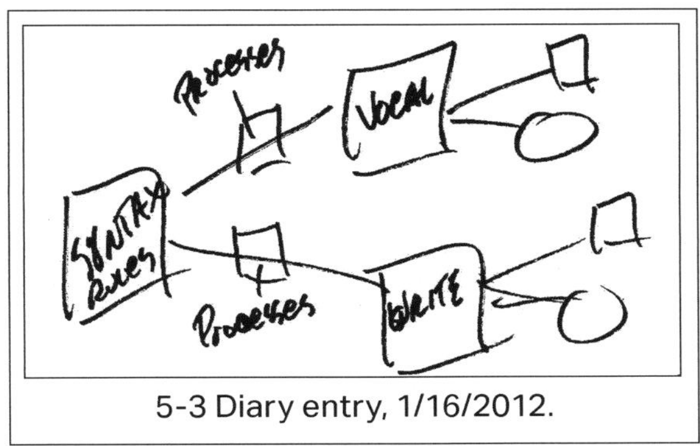

5-3 Diary entry, 1/16/2012.

Since my speech was doing so well and my writing was so bad, I thought there had to be different syntaxes. On a walk, I reviewed the scenario. I knew the definition of "syntax." It is the rules of sentence structure and language. With two modalities with such different problems (in terms of their deficits), I thought there must have been two syntaxes, one for speaking and one for writing.

As I thought about it for a while, I figured each one had to have its own syntax. Under normal conditions, the product of each modality would have been identical. With a disease like aphasia, language products were demonstrably damaged differently from each other. With two syntaxes (I even thought there might be more), I figured each individual syntax must be fed by a "master" syntax. Those individual syntaxes had to be cloned. Then, each clone was damaged in its own way.

After several more days of thinking, I came to a new realization. There could not have been two syntaxes. There can only be one. I had been thinking about how difficult it would be to create identical syntaxes, each with its own defects. Then each damaged syntax got better in its own way. I had been drawing a picture in my mind of the "master" syntax with individual syntaxes drawn from it, and then each modality being drawn from *that*. It was getting too hard. As a result of thinking along that line, I realized there must be only one source from which all modalities must draw for language sustenance. At that point, I changed my drawing to indicate that the damage must have been "downstream" from each modality, not above it (figure 5-3). Each modality drew its language and rules from the one-and-only syntax. Each modality was damaged in its own way.

Aphasia Mountain

I drew a metaphorical picture of a mountain range with the letters from the word "APHASIA" written across the peaks (figure 5-4). Since I could not write, I had been using many metaphorical drawings about what I was thinking. Every day I thought about what had happened to me. In my metaphorical mountain peaks, I had a sense that each letter had rolled down one side or the other of the "Great Divide." I realized the cells were likely destroyed at random.

I also realized that the brain circuits had to have been redundant. Otherwise there would have been an On/Off switch with On (OK) and Off (not OK). There was plenty of damage, yet I was still able to "see" most of the letters. The deficits of one letter or another were presented in different modalities. Some were fine and others were damaged. Those that were damaged were still not damaged enough to have lost all of their influence. The alphabet list in my diary showed 13 letters were fine and 13 were damaged. I reviewed my alphabet list several times throughout my dairy; it was still 13 "good" and 13 "bad" letters. (*They weren't bad, they were drawn that way!*)

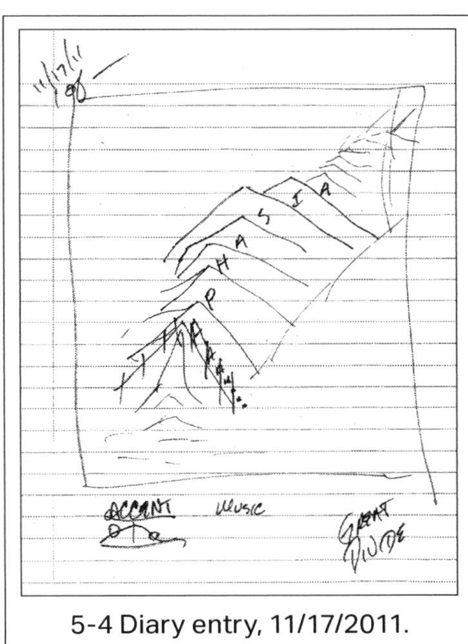

5-4 Diary entry, 11/17/2011.

It was an interesting problem. I thought about the letters and their damage. I thought about the letters within the context of the different modalities. I thought each modality was redundant at the system level. Each letter was redundant at the cell-network level. I imagined there wasn't just one mountain. There had to be a chain of mountains, each with its own slope. Some had been downgraded from a mountain to a hill. Others hardly lost their grade. There wasn't any hill I went up that didn't come down a mountain. Some problems were confronted by deep ravines and steep peaks. The mind can challenge even the highest peaks. Problem solving is one instrument of an enriched toolkit designed to learn.

CHAPTER SIX

METAPHOR IS THERAPY

Metaphors may create realities for us, especially social realities. A metaphor may thus be a guide for future action. Such actions will, of corse, fit the metaphor. This will, in turn, reinforce the power of the metaphor to make experience coherent. In this sense metaphors can be self-fulfilling prophecies.

—George Lakoff and Mark Johnson,
Metaphors We Live By

The metaphor is a figure of speech that compares one thing to another different (but similar) idea. Metaphors look for the hidden similarities between them. I used metaphors throughout my diary. The first segment of my diary used metaphorical pictures and diagrams. Since I could not explain my deficits using any language you might know, I used metaphors (and metaphorical drawings) to help me understand my deficits.

Metaphors are not right or wrong per se. Sometimes a metaphor doesn't provide the right emphasis or approach about the lesson. Sometimes a metaphor doesn't provide enough history or background to explain the moral. The metaphors rattling around in my head gave me a sense of how my mind was working. I imagined (assumed, wished, thought of) any number of metaphors I hoped would help me understand what was wrong with my language and how I could fix it. I used the brain as the target, metaphorically speaking.

I could think, but couldn't explain in writing what I was thinking. So in the absence of nonsense writing, metaphorical drawings explained what I was thinking.

Each metaphor contributed, in its own way, a small measure of understanding. In the beginning I was unaware of so many things; every idea, thought, drawing, and metaphor must have soaked into my brain unconsciously. I didn't employ metaphors on purpose. The metaphor is a tool built for learning. No one told (assigned, persuaded, convinced) me to write a metaphor or consider a metaphor. It seemed metaphors *existed* within a unique portion of my memory. As I considered my problems, metaphorical explanations appeared like unbidden guests. A metaphor can provide a therapeutic explanation without your being consciously aware of that effect. No one can *instruct* a patient to *use* metaphors. A therapist will love you for using them, though. It does take more time to comb through your memory looking for a particular *A* with similar *B* ideas. A person with aphasia (PWA) can still learn from both an *A* and a *B* even if they themselves are damaged. A patient can combine their past with their current deficits to build a new reconstructed "you." Metaphor is therapy.

Gamma Knife®

A friend of mine discovered he had brain tumors. Within weeks the doctors told him a Gamma Knife® procedure was required to help constrain the growth of the tumors. He told me about it, and I looked it up on Google (figure 6-1). The Gamma Knife® directs high-intensity radiation therapy concentrated on a small target point in the brain. The device is placed in a circular array on a specialized helmet directing each source of the radiation at the target.

Using a Gamma Knife® metaphor, the metaphor therapy "lenses" the therapeutic energy (radiation) towards a certain (metaphorically speaking) target. The source of the energy is experience-dependent activities. Using metraphors provides an additional therapeutic premium from a number of sources (reading, writing, speaking), directed at the target. In this case, the target is the brain that activates plasticity to rebuild the networks.

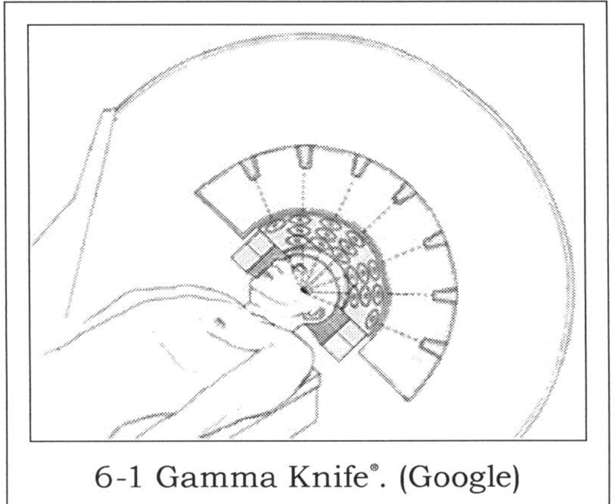

6-1 Gamma Knife®. (Google)

Each of the sources contributed their own therapeutic measure, including my diary, recording my voice, taking pictures, and reading. Additional "radiation" sources (metaphors) were arrayed to provide a magnifier effect. Therapeutic activities power the brain. Thinking is the accelerant.

Message Rock

Early pioneers used "message rocks" or "writing rocks" along the trails heading out west (figure 6-2). They inscribed their names, dates, and messages (no iPhones back then) to signal family and friends where they were and what was coming next. It appears I left messages for (and about) myself in the future. These messages were left without grammar.

Real words appeared in sentence-like structures. There had to have been *some* intelligence in the entries, but they were without meaning. Earlier pages in my diary might as well have been pictures on a cave—like an archeologist tries to extract meaning from pictures and diagrams without much to go on. I had been trying to understand what I was thinking, using pictures to convey what I otherwise couldn't do with words. There was another important discovery in the "message rocks." It turned out not all of my language was damaged. Math and numeracy communications appeared to be functioning fine. Many of my "message rocks" (graphs, charts, and drawings) made pictures make sense. Of course, it was a picture without the thousand words I would have preferred. Yet, it was a start.

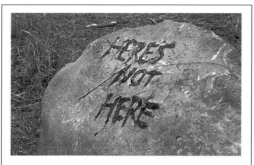

6-2 Message rocks. (Wikipedia)

Photosynthesis

Photosynthesis is a process using leaves to convert sunlight into energy (figure 6-3). The plants and leaves contain light-dependent reactions that provide almost all of the energy required to sustain life on earth.

The leaves change sunlight into chemical energy (usually sugar) and give off oxygen (amazingly) as a waste product. I had always wondered about the process of photosynthesis. We learned about it in elementary school. As we got older, we knew it without really understanding it. We all remember the concept. If you are like me, we are always amazed that so much of the world comes from just sunlight. Sunlight drives pretty much everything. I had never thought about photosynthesis in my life until I had my stroke. Photosynthesis was a miracle metaphor!

As I got better, I read more about the process of how a brain works. In theory, I know how the brain works. Like photosynthesis, I knew it without really knowing it. I had learned about the brain and its capacity to change and be altered, based on plasticity. The full term is called *experience-dependent neural plasticity*. The process *converts thinking* (it might as well be sunlight) into chemical and electrical energy. As soon as I read about plasticity, I realized photosynthesis is a similar process. Plasticity converts the process of thinking, problem solving, and metaphors into learning, memory, and language.

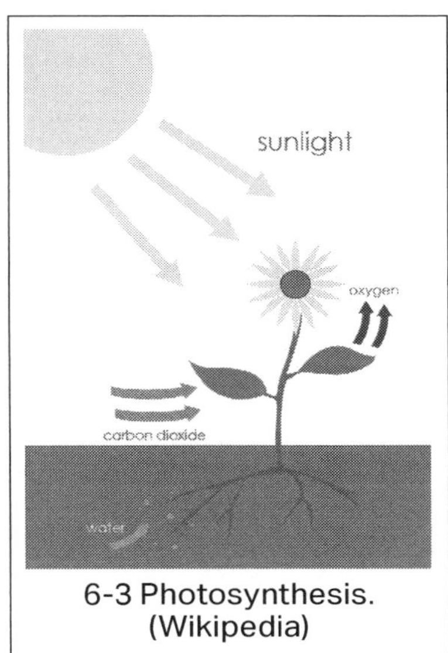

6-3 Photosynthesis. (Wikipedia)

CHAPTER SEVEN

EVIDENCE MATTERS

Believe that life is worth living and your belief will help create the fact.

—William James

Diary

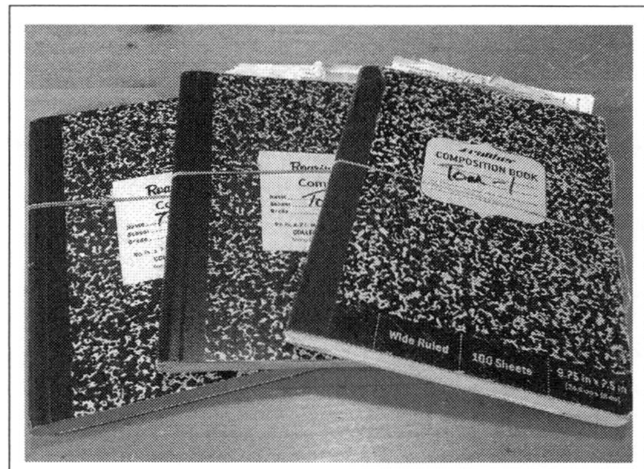

7-1 Original composition books, 10/27/2011.

I wrote without knowing that what I was writing was wrong. I wrote the first entry in my diary shortly after my first therapy session (figure 7-1). There was no grammar or syntax, yet all the words were real words. Amazingly enough, I misspelled a word within that paragraph, lined it out, and *fixed it* and it *still* made no sense. As days and weeks went by, my diary continued to look "fine." I was completely unaware of what I had done. And I kept doing it for 500 pages.

My "stories" in my diary were hardly stories. They were snippets and glimpses of meaning. They came in the form of pictures, drawings, images, graphs, tables, and writing. Since I could not understand what had happened to my brain, recording everything seemed to be the next best thing to understanding what I meant.

My diary was a message in a bottle. It became its own metaphor. I wrote what I thought was a diary, not unlike Anne Frank's diary. I thought it would help to describe my stroke events for others to see. I didn't realize my diary would be something a reader could not read, or make sense of. I wrote in it almost every day. I added the date, day, and often the time and place. I described my problems. I wrote about the details of one deficit or another. Just like any diary.

However, I didn't know I couldn't write in any reasonable way. I was unaware of the contents of what I was saying. Eventually I was able to see it for what it was. When I "saw" it for the first time, I could see how bad my "eyes" had been. Despite this, my diary was still useful. I understood a lot more of my deficits as a result of seeing my thoughts through metaphors, graphs, and charts.

Messages have been put into bottles since ancient times. Messages were sent with the hope they would be found, and with all kinds of reasons including romantic, scientific, and for the purposes of war. The first recorded messages in bottles were released around 310 BC, by the ancient Greek philosopher Theophrastus, as part of an experiment to show the Mediterranean Sea was formed by the inflowing Atlantic Ocean.

During his return to Spain, following his first voyage to the New World, Christopher Columbus threw a report of his discovery in a sealed cask, along with a note asking it to be passed on to the queen. He hoped the news would make it back even if he did not survive. In fact, Columbus survived, and the cask did not.

In the 16th century, the English navy used bottle messages to send information ashore about enemy positions. Queen Elizabeth I created an official position of "Uncorker of Ocean Bottles" in case anyone else opened a bottle containing secret messages. They could face the death penalty! I was the only "uncorker" for my own bottle. It wasn't a secret, but I never showed my diary to anyone—not my therapist or my family—until after I published my first book.

Voice Recording

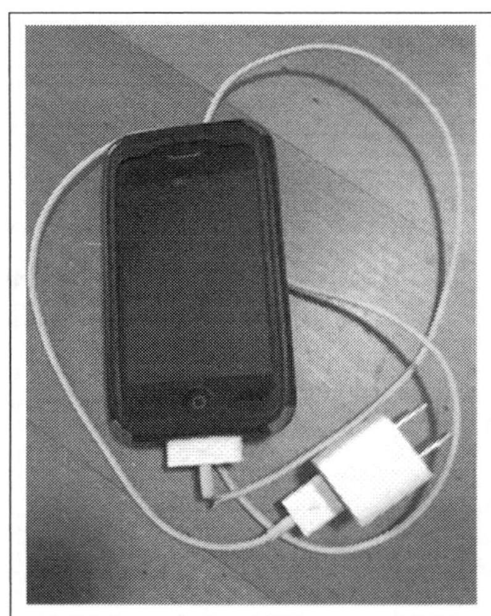

7-2 My original iPhone, 2011.

I don't know why I started to record myself (figure 7-2). As it was my habit, I had been walking every day. I always talked to myself while walking; I had always considered it the best way to think through a problem. In this case, I struggled with a problem I still couldn't identify. Talking to myself seemed to help. It was soothing to (mentally) review my problems (not that I knew what they were) and the solutions (again, solutions for problems I was still unable to define). Eventually, speaking out loud (and recording) became new tools. I walked for miles while thinking about my problems. I tallied my mileage in my calendar, starting on Tuesday, October 11, 2011. I do remember being told about the possibility of getting lost and to be careful. I walked 135 miles before I started to record myself on Friday, November 4, 2011. I must have been talking to myself the entire time. With all that walking and talking there must have been an indication I was thinking ... about something. What was I thinking?

I couldn't study the problems without some physical artifact of what might have been my thinking. My first recording was the beginning of the proof. All that walking must have alerted me. I needed to listen to what I had been saying the week before or the day before or the minute before. I had been saying things (literally, talking out loud) for a month before I realized I needed to hear what I had been saying. I had to *understand* what I had been saying. Without recording myself, I couldn't understand much. I *couldn't* study what I *couldn't* understand if I *couldn't* record it. The recordings told the tale.

I recorded each clip along the walk and then played them back immediately. I usually listened once and then moved on to the next recording. Often, the next recording was connected to whatever I had been thinking previously. If I had a question in one recording, I reflected on what I had said and commented again in the next clip. After listening once, I typically did not play them again. I saved all the files and had them transcribed years later for my first book. It had been years since I listened to my first recording, and I listened to all of

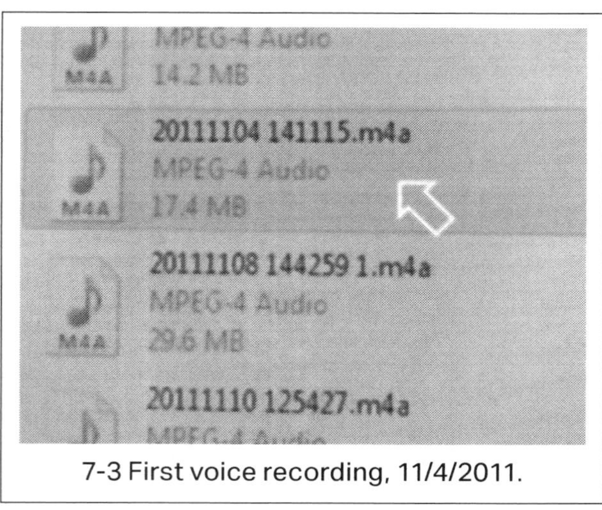

7-3 First voice recording, 11/4/2011.

them. The first one was a perfect example of my deficits, *spoken in the moment*, crystallized on tape for future scientists (and stroke survivors) to see.

The first recording was a microcosm of my impaired language. Previously, I have mentioned the automatics. While working with my daughter and again with my therapist, I realized I could say the numbers in sequence but could not find the one number I needed to say.

The *first* sentence of my *first* recording presented me with the first physical evidence about this deficit *and* I was aware of it in the moment.

> *Mom [my wife, Laura] going to work the whole time because I couldn't remember anything; went to sleep and woke up about around 1 o'clock ... 1-2-3-4-5-6-7-8-9 ... 9 ... 9 AM this morning and that is when I couldn't find out that Mom's had gone ... I never had lost it* (Figure 7-3).

While talking to myself, I *knew* I had gotten up that morning. But instead, I said "*1 o'clock.*" As soon as I could say it, I could *tell* it was wrong. (It was still me. I wasn't delusional. I didn't make a mistake on purpose.) I was talking into my iPhone and as soon as I could hear it, I could *tell* I didn't want to say "*1 o'clock.*" But I had said it anyway. I immediately used the sequence of "*1, 2, 3...*" and arrived at the number 9. I had woken up at 9:00 AM that morning. I had made a mistake. I was aware of the mistake. That was a good thing. Finding a mistake, seeing a mistake, and correcting a mistake all fit the mold of awareness. Not all mistakes can be found. Or at least not until more evidence is revealed.

For example, I was aware of the "empty word" problem. But not in the same way my therapist had indicated. When I spoke with my therapist and I couldn't say what I wanted to say, I would use (and I remembered saying it) "empty" words or words without content. At least to me, they made sense. When I couldn't name an object or an item, I would say "the thing" or "that thing." I could feel the (real) tension in my mind of *not* being able to say the word, and I used (as fast as I could) an easy word that meant (in my mind) what I *intended it to be*. That was me on the inside.

On the outside, my therapist *knew* I couldn't say what I was trying to say. She noted I was using "empty words." She didn't know the "empty words" I used *meant* the item or object which appeared in my mind. Yes, I could *see* it in my mind. However, I couldn't grab it in time to *say* it in a normal conversation. As a result, I used an easier word. An *easier* word for people with aphasia usually means the "empty words" (*thing, that, something*, and others), or "plug" words. They can be used in the course of a conversation when the right words can't be found *in time*. As a result, an often-used word can be plugged in for now. Many people with aphasia use the aphorism, "We can *see* it but we can't *say* it." We can indicate it in our minds. We can (mentally) point at whatever the item might be, knowing what it is, and still say, "I know what that is ... that ... *thing*."

My therapist talked about paraphasias and neologisms in my first assessment. I did not know what the words meant *then*. I hardly understand them *now*. I have read the definitions, so I understand what they are meant to be. As I recorded myself, many examples of paraphasias and neologisms appeared in my speech. I listened to my recordings once or twice, but not enough to perceive the substituting of words for what I wanted to say.

I had said: "I wrote a bunch of stuff in my lawyer." Clearly I probably meant "diary" instead of "lawyer." I never knew I had said it *even after I listened to myself* on the recording. It wasn't until *after I had my tapes transcribed* that I saw, for the first time, words that were clearly wrong.

It was great to know my therapist had heard *me* say "panger" for pencil and "blesker" for whistle. I would not *know* what I had said unless the therapist told me.

My son told me later that I had said "airport" instead of "hospital" while he drove me home *from the hospital*. Without recording myself on a regular basis, I never would have known what I was saying. That is not to say I understood everything I heard on the tapes, either. There was enough evidence in my recordings to make me *more* aware of my speaking. Being *more* aware isn't the same as being *completely* aware. It was interesting (to me, anyway) when I caught (and was conscious of) one error or another. I didn't *find* those errors as much as I *stumbled* over them and I didn't stumble on purpose. "Stumbling" seemed to be part of recovery. Not unlike stubbing a toe, I could *feel* it … in the same way I could *feel* an error. I couldn't find it. I couldn't describe it. I could *hear* my mistakes, but only if I recorded my voice. <u>It was one more aspect of learning through evidence.</u>

I used what I called "Voice Memos" in my iPhone for almost two years. The first 11 months of recordings were all transcribed and appeared in my first book. There were 144 voice memos, with an average of four minutes each, from November 2011 until July 2012. The total time of the voice memos contained over 10 hours of my voice rendered in four- to five-minute segments. *If I had not recorded myself, I would not be who I am today.*

My recovery must have arrived from many different directions. My therapist was an important part of my recovery. Most of my recovery came as a result of practicing reading, writing, and speaking. My brain must have been thinking about my problems every single day. That is what it does. It thinks. My brain was thinking what it would take to get better while *keeping track* of my experiences.

Since I spent a lot of my time walking while talking to myself, as mentioned before, I recorded myself. I had also been silently reading from my computer. I had had a hard time actually reading from a book. I can't explain why. I just knew. It was frustrating. It was annoying. It bothered me the same way a mosquito bothers me at a picnic. Except this was a swarm of bother.

As a result, I did not even try to read a book for a while. I figured it would resolve itself at some point. I knew I could read words, and I figured it would take time. I started recording myself reading a book and thought it might help. This page was recorded on December 28, 2011. As I had noted, this passage said: *"Reading it was really, really terrible."* I was glad to have found a professional transcriber with verbatim recording-transcribing skills. If I had not, I would *never* have known how bad it was. Again, feedback was important at every level. Still, I didn't record too many books, and those I read aloud were awful. They were so awful as to be funny, which you can see in this paragraph (sorry for the profanity!).

> *The controvers-, promp-, the controbutual, constibutional l-l-lane, r-r-row of a language in relation to thought is not to suppor-, to suppor the m-, the m-, the material phonetics, mening by which ideas mess be expressed. It is to act as intermedior between thought and sound in such a way that the combination of both necessarily produce a ma-ma-mator-matorially puh-pum- (interjects, 'Ha-ha') matorially compotilly duladalis (laughs) of the units (interjects, 'Oh, shit')*

thought corructic by nature is made frecisely by this, by this process of salimentation. And what happens is neither a signfulmation, a signfulmation of thoughts into me-metter-m-metter, nor a fonsonation of signs into ideas. What becomes in a somewhat mysterial process is thought, is by thought/sound evolving de-devetions and in a, an in language takes shape from its lintwistically u-u-units in between those two amorphicus message. Mun nite think of it as being like air in contract with water, in contract, contract with water. Changes in appervarial, apperveriable pressure breaks up the sentence of the water in series on divisions, meaning label, labels, ways. The correlation between thought and sound and the relition of the two is like that. (Voice memo, 12/28/2011)

I continued to record and talk to myself while walking. It seemed to me that talking to myself was the equivalent of thinking *about* what I was thinking. I thought while I talked, and I talked while I thought. For all the time spent, I only recorded a small amount of my thinking. The rest of the time I continued to think with every step. The act of walking must have been the lubricant for thought. As I walked, I thought about different aspects of my deficits. I had been considering how it was that each of my damaged modalities was so different from the other. How could that be? I could *tell* my speaking was doing well and my writing was awful. I needed more evidence. Voice recording provided part of it. My diary provided more.

Photographs

I took pictures before I knew what I was doing. I don't know why I started taking pictures, but later I was glad I did. I took

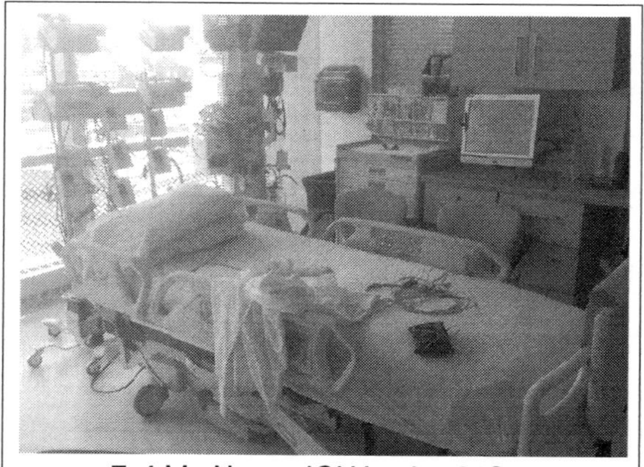

7-4 My Neuro ICU bed at MGH, Wednesday, 9/28/11.

five pictures during the entire time at the hospital (figure 7-4, 7-5, 7-6, 7-7, 7-8). I didn't remember any of them. Truth be told, I didn't know about the pictures until I found them in Florida, a year later—and I was baffled. I looked at those pictures and had no memory of having taken them. But they had to be mine. I had downloaded my iPhone pictures to my computer and there they were. Then I looked at the JPEG label for the pictures and found the date and time of each one. It was the first time I realized that memory can be a problem. Without the evidence, I wouldn't have known about the problem.

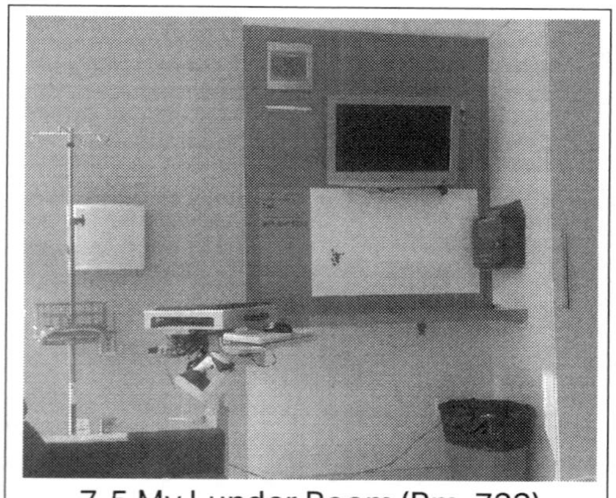

7-5 My Lunder Room (Rm. 732) at MGH, Wednesday, 9/28/11.

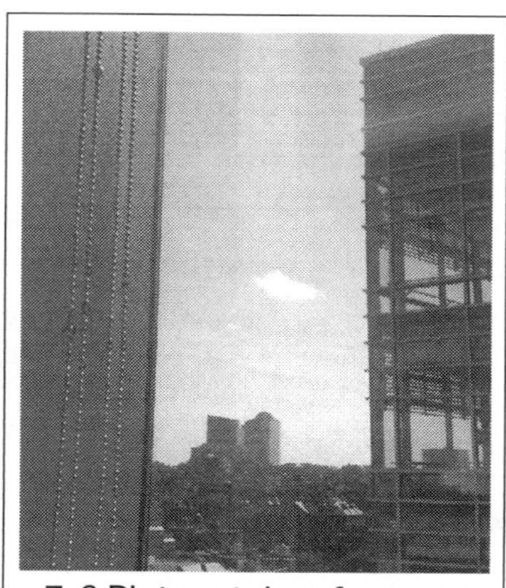

7-6 Picture taken from my room at MGH, Friday, 9/30/11.

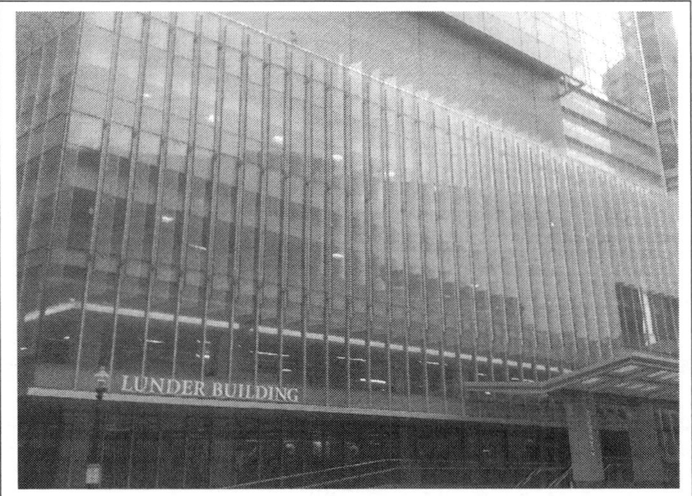

7-7 Leaving the Lunder Building, MGH, Saturday, 10/1/11.

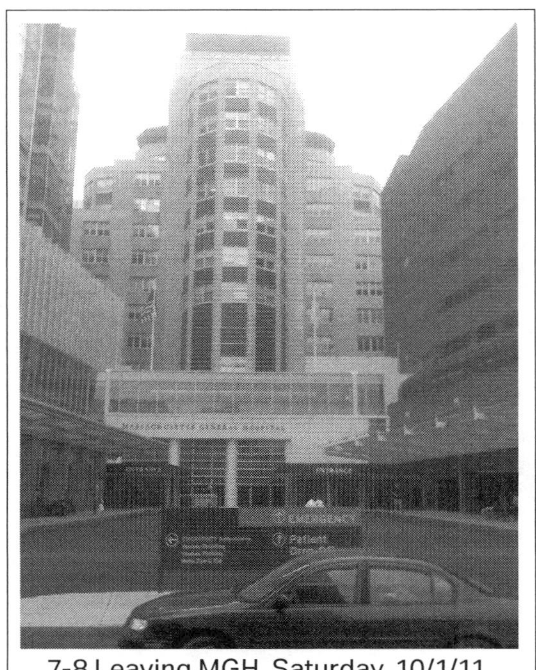

7-8 Leaving MGH, Saturday, 10/1/11.

The next two pictures in my iPhone were taken *eight days later*. I left the hospital on Saturday, October 1, 2011. I *thought* I had taken those two pictures on the next day, what would have been Sunday, October 2, 2011. It wasn't until later that I saw the pictures in Florida and noticed the dates for the first time. I found those two "walking farm" pictures. They were taken on Sunday, October 9, 2011, *eight days later* (figures 7-9, 7-10).

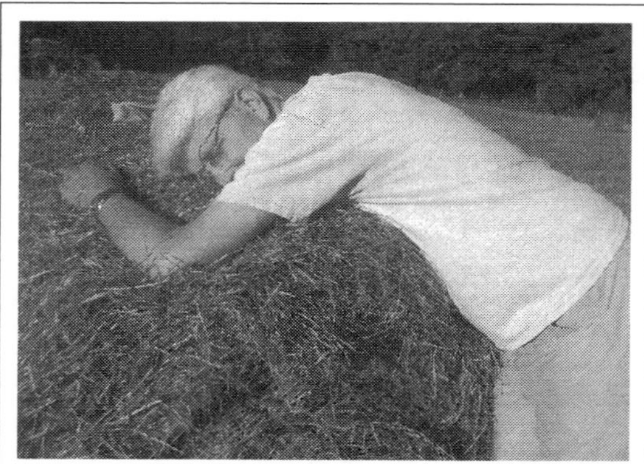

7-9 Walking Farm, Sunday, 10/09/11

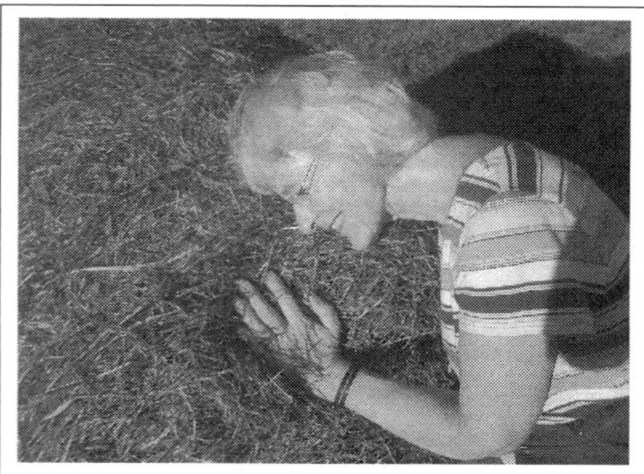

7-10 Walking Farm, Sunday, 10/09/11

You can see why taking pictures (or videos) is so important. I didn't know much about my memory or that part of my deficits related to memory. The seven pictures were so helpful. I took only seven pictures during those two weeks. So it wasn't much. But what if I had not taken *any* pictures? My memory at the time was already fractured. At least, having the pictures (whether I was conscious of taking them or not) provided the evidence that *someday* they would provide me with more facts. You will often have memory problems as a result of a brain injury. Creating physical evidence (a diary, audio recordings, pictures, and videos) can provide an external hard drive that can save your (real but unaware) memories until you can access them later, as your brain gets better.

Evidence (diary, recordings, and pictures) provided the proof of what I was thinking. I'm sure I would have been thinking even without my evidence. Aphasia is a mystery. You can't figure it out without some clues. If I didn't have those clues, I don't know how long it would have taken to crack the code. Keeping track of every modality provided the clues to recovery. Evidence matters.

CHAPTER EIGHT
FEEDBACK MATTERS

My thinking is first and last and always for the sake of my doing.
—William James

I remember being told that "awareness of deficits" was important for recovery. I noted that term without being sure what it meant. It appeared in my prognosis that I was "aware" (as told by my therapist) of my deficits. I had been thinking (considering, wondering, questioning) about that sentence for a long time. Partly because I was aware (of my deficits). Partly because I wasn't aware (of being aware) of my deficits.

I had been thinking about the *idea* of being aware. I considered there had to be a sequence of events *ending* with being aware. What were the earlier steps approaching (yet not reaching) awareness? I looked for the proximate steps to awareness and realized *feedback* was needed *before* awareness. *Evidence* was needed before *that*. I realized that I had to go back before I could go forward. I started with *evidence*, then *feedback*, and then discovered *awareness*. Awareness doesn't appear on its own. It doesn't start without more data and more feedback. The meaning of feedback includes:

> *... conceptualized as information provided by an agent (e.g., teacher, peer, book, parent, self, experience) regarding aspects of one's performance or understanding. A teacher or parent can provide corrective information, a peer can provide an alternative strategy, a book can provide information to clarify ideas, a parent can provide encouragement, and a learner can look up the answer to evaluate the correctness of a response. Feedback thus is a "consequence" of performance* (Hattie and Timperley).

The consequence of my performance would not have existed without the feedback. Without keeping track of my performance I would not have had the needed feedback. A speech therapist can provide some amount of secondhand feedback. But it is not the same and does not provide the therapeutic energy (punch, drive, oomph) required to increase plasticity and learning.

My research found several (about 20) intensive aphasia programs in the country. Many programs with the title "intensive therapy" provide more practice with reading, writing, speaking, and listening. The programs usually consist of about 30 hours per week, for four to six weeks. Each day is spent with different therapists and different activities related to one modality or another. To the degree there are more "intensive" activities, most of them use the same activities as before, only more intensive, which is to say, more time and more "doses."

Each report provided a limited kind of feedback. As my formal therapy progressed, I had also started keeping my diary and recording my voice. As time went by, I was starting to tell that even though my formal "grades" were "going up," I still couldn't write worth a damn.

I wanted the feedback from the therapist's report. I also needed continuous feedback. In order to get that kind of feedback, you need continuous communication. The only feedback I got from my therapist was from our "communicating" 45 minutes about my deficits, twice a week. My therapist made notes about me and my experience. I got to review them eventually. They were delivered in too-big-to-use chunks of information. They were too big and they came too late. Every time I spoke, read, or wrote in the course of everyday living, I needed the feedback that life provided.

All of my (therapeutic) activities were bundled in neural feedback. It was OK that I didn't do well. But poorly or not, the brain provides internal feedback over and above any feedback I could consciously absorb from formal therapy and short reports. My brain could compare the difference between what was right and what was wrong, *without* being conscious of it.

The activities of the brain "flow" at billions of flows per second. Those flows contain the active ingredients (in the form of experience) required to activate plasticity. The reports from my therapist came twice a week in condensed, objective feedback.

I myself provided intensive activities (writing, reading, speaking, walking) and immediate experience-dependent data in real time. If doses from *conventional* therapy provided x therapy energy units, then my own *enriched and intensive* therapy was 10x (or 100x) the therapy energy units. Recovery from aphasia is always about *the doing.* Yet it is more about the *right kind of doing* (enriched, multi-functional, evidence-based) and the *right kind of "doses"* (immediate, real-time, interactive).

CHAPTER NINE
AWARENESS MATTERS

The mind has become aware of itself.
—Ralph Waldo Emerson

When did I become aware of my stroke? I was out in the street when it happened. I remember looking at my shoe, staring at it—and that was it. I couldn't see, hear, or walk. I appeared in a chair at the pharmacy at CVS in Waltham, MA. I wasn't aware of anything between the street and the chair. It felt like I woke up from a deep sleep.

I looked around and saw people in front of me. I couldn't tell who they were. I was awake (aware) enough to realize I was in the chair. I could tell my right arm kept drooping. I could see it dangling, on its own, without my having any idea what it was doing or even if it was mine. I picked it up and put it back on my lap. Every once in a while it dropped again and I went to get it. It felt like a dog with a stick. I wasn't conscious enough to comment whether it was a stick or an arm. Everything was moving in slow motion (if things were hardly moving at all). Every time I retrieved my arm, I brushed my pants as if there was lint on them. I think I was worried about being dirty. I remember remembering with a less-than-normal consciousness.

I didn't know what happened next, but I was no longer in the chair. I woke up again. This time I was in a gurney, with EMTs on either side of me. Apparently, I drifted away ... not asleep but not awake, either. The EMTs must have lifted me onto the stretcher, and I became more aware then. I was still in no condition to understand what had happened. The EMTs were talking about something. I didn't know what it was. The EMT on my left was comforting me (as far as I could tell). I could see him.

The EMT on the right was strapping me in. I could feel the stretcher rocking. I couldn't see him at the time. I figured he was behind me. He was so close, I could feel his breath on my face.

A hand appeared out of nowhere. It was only a hand, no body. It was pulling the seat belt. It disappeared in a second. It happened again and disappeared just as quickly. I recognized something different (bad, strange, odd) had happened. I couldn't define it or express it. My body told me something was wrong. At that point, a head appeared. It was a head and it floated right in front of me, like a balloon with a beard, on a string. I was sure I looked at him for less than a second. The appearance of the two hands and the discombobulated head confirmed, without any conscious appreciation, that something was wrong.

I drifted away again and didn't come back until I was at MGH in the ER. The nurse was infusing me with tPA. Almost immediately I could hear something like popcorn popping in my brain. That was the tPA dissolving my blood clot.

They sent me to my Neuro ICU room at about 3:00 AM on Tuesday morning. I stayed there for a day and a half, until they moved me to a new room on Wednesday afternoon. I have no memory from the time at ER until I was moved. That is not to say that nothing happened. I was a part of the experience, but I have no memory of it.

A speech-language pathologist (SLP) conducted an assessment on Wednesday morning, before I was transferred to my new room. Even though I couldn't remember it, the assessment said it all.

> *Cog.: Alert, oriented, focused and attentive. Social pragmatics within normal limits (WNL). Demonstrates insight into deficits and emerging understanding of the implications of his new disabilities.*

I didn't see the report for years. I didn't get a copy of it at the hospital, and didn't know what it was, anyway. When I got to Florida I ordered all my reports from the hospital. If I hadn't done that, I would never have read them. After my stroke and for some amount of time, I couldn't remember things that evidence showed otherwise. Reading this report, it seemed that I was "Alert, oriented, focused and attentive." Interesting. I was not aware of it. On the same day, I (apparently) talked with my wife and told her I was seeing the therapist as well. I would not have known what I had said, except for an email (collected years later) from my wife, telling the kids about it.

I was healthy (as far as I knew). I walked around the hospital. I watched and pointed and observed and thought. Apparently, short-term memory appeared to be incredibly short. So much of "me" was still ... *not* me. Not entirely. It is interesting to read the report *now*, after realizing I actually said those things. I was not aware of my deficits in any conscious way. I didn't realize the various levels of consciousness. My problems with short-term memory confused my reality. It took a long time before I realized there was a difference between my performance and my *awareness* of my performance. The therapist witnessed what appeared to be an "attentive" patient.

Only now can I say I am glad that I was alert and attentive. Because at the time, there was a rupture between being *consciously* aware and being *unaware* yet still conscious. I was variously unaware in the course of my 11-month recovery. Like a slow leak in a tire, you can drive a car for a long time before it goes flat. I leaked awareness. As the therapist said, the report was indicative of my aptitude, but without being conscious of it. As the saying goes: The light was on, but no one was home.

The hospital discharged me for the next stage at home. I was the same actor in a new play. But I couldn't remember my lines. Literally. I was unaware of my performance. An invisible cloak separated *me* from a *more conscious* me. I could *think* on one side, but couldn't read, write, or speak well on the other. It was not unlike the EMT who I couldn't see. I knew he was there. I could *feel* him. But like a ghost, he only appeared every once in a while.

I didn't know what it might take to break the cypher. I wasn't consciously aware of any of the tools that might be needed. Metaphors inferred meaning when there was otherwise no meaning to see. I had been keeping track with my diary. I used metaphorical drawings to explain what I was unable to say. It was the beginning of smoke. Fire broke out later.

I had problems with my language. While speaking, I could transpose one bad (inappropriate, unsuitable, wrong) word instead of another. While writing, I wrote page after page using real words, but without any meaning. While reading, I could understand individual words, but if coupled together they didn't make sense. While listening, I heard some words, but still couldn't hear what they meant.

Each modality had its own local deficit with its own "personality." For example, I had thought I "lost my grammar."

I assumed I had lost my grammar in *every* modality. Each deficit was different. Writing and reading were bad. Speaking and listening, although damaged in their own way, were still largely intact. At the beginning I had been thinking that *all* modalities were damaged badly and in the same way. I was unaware of the composition and severity of each of the individual deficits. I remained unaware until more evidence presented itself.

Metaphorical drawings provided the evidence of my thinking throughout my diary. I drew some (pretty good) pictures of boxcars. I drew in three dimensions, three cars including the wheels. I didn't draw the couplings. I did that on purpose. There were gaps with vertical lines between each car, and arrows pointing at the gaps indicated the couplings were *not* there. The caption read:

> *Cloak, believe want to book to curious serious in the chemistry in brain. See you send sentence you expanding you again thank see before.*
> (Diary, 11/2/2011)

I still don't know what I was saying in that passage. I could tell from the pictures that I was describing the problem. The rules of grammar were gone. No one had told me about it. I could tell that the couplings used to connect words were gone.

It's too bad there isn't a mental recorder. I wish I had been able to record my thoughts using the grammar I now know I didn't have. If I *did* have the capacity (the capacity to capture everything in my brain, even though damaged) to recover everything perfectly, I would have been able to explain to you about my errant boxcars.

In the absence of some neurological miracle, my diary and all the devices that recorded my erstwhile thoughts provided an imperfect yet still sufficient description of what it means to "lose your language" from aphasia. I discovered many shades of awareness of my deficits. This was one of them. Awareness was the *primus inter pares* (first among equals) of my deficits.

Part 3

The Principles of Plasticity in Action

PART 3 INTRODUCTION

All of the principles of experience-dependent neural plasticity were grounded in experience (doing, practicing, making, understanding). I had never heard of the word "plasticity" before. The principles (values, beliefs, philosophies) of the experience-dependent component of plasticity *depended* on the act of experience without my being aware of the *need*.

I was given a prescription for speech therapy. That was the only activity I had been *told* (instructed, stated, communicated) to do. It was the first experience-dependent activity, but not the last. Within weeks I had initiated all kinds of new therapies. I kept my diary. I recorded myself. I took pictures of the world around me. I participated in all those things without being aware of the need. Having said that, I believe my brain was neurologically in need of the activities that would feed the need. I was not consciously aware of the need (impetus, motivation, drive) to assign experience-dependent activities designed to satisfy neurological needs borne by my aphasia deficits.

But there was a need to adjust to the new reality of my stroke. I wasn't conscious of it. My brain instructed me to start working with as many different activities as I could find. In my brain, it was pleasing (like scratching an itch) every time I could notice a (mental) irritation.

I didn't go in search of finding one particular kind of activity to address one particular kind of plasticity principle.

I conducted every possible kind of activity. Each of those activities provided an amalgamation of the principles of plasticity. It is only in retrospect that scientists can single out one principle or another that can be applied to one experience or another. In my case, I used examples of different experiences that tended to lean on one principle or another. I am sure all my experiences were engaged with all the principles of plasticity at one degree or another.

Here are some examples of my deficits, my therapeutic activities, and the principles of plasticity. In many cases I was not fully aware of one deficit or another (and what it would take to fix them) until after the deficit revealed itself. Sometimes those deficits didn't appear for months or years. That's not to say the deficits weren't there. Being unaware that a deficit has existed for a while still gives the appearance of not having the deficit—until it appears.

There was a continuum of awareness. Being *unaware* of a deficit is one thing. Being unaware of how to *fix it* is another. Being unaware of the neurological principles of plasticity is another component in the problem-solving equation. All of my activities created additional plasticity. The challenge of recovery is to create as many enriched and learning environments as possible, where the brain can perform its magic.

CHAPTER TEN

USE IT OR LOSE IT

Because it is a use-it-or-lose-it brain, when we develop a map area (in the brain), we long to keep it activated. Just as our muscles become impatient for exercise if we've been sitting all day ….

—Norman Doidge
The Brain That Changes Itself

I had been working hard on my deficits for almost two years. I didn't realize some portions of my deficits were still untouched, therapeutic-wise. Public speaking and executive function deficits were among them. I didn't know it at the time. I assumed that public speaking was a natural skill and not one I had to worry about. And I had no idea about executive function. It is described as someone with hyperactivity and chronic problems with assigning daily tasks. So, I didn't think about it until it was (almost) too late. This was certainly one skill that had atrophied. It was a deficit not yet in evidence to me. As a result, I was unaware it had decayed. My treatment would have to be tailored. The "use it or lose it" maxim seemed to fit. I had to start using my public speaking or risk losing it forever.

Public Speaking (and Executive Function)

After I moved to Florida, I continued to practice my language. I knew I'd have to get a job at some point. I was a volunteer at Flagler Hospital. Plus I volunteered at a local high school, teaching two classes: Business Academy in Business Ownership, and Principles of Entrepreneurship. It was my first time speaking in public since my stroke. There had not been any opportunity to speak therapeutically in Boston. I had always been a public speaker, so I was concerned about getting it right. I started my classes in January 2013.

I figured the best thing I could do was practice with students. I had two classes: one in the afternoon and one 45-minute class, with lunch wedged in the middle of the class.

I developed materials in advance. I organized the classes by groups, with their own activities. Then each group would discuss their ideas with the rest of the class. There were always some students with their own emotional issues (hating lunch, hating the group, or hating talking). The classes did go well, all things considered.

I could see lingering problems of mine that weren't fully corrected. I had word-finding problems in front of the class. I forgot some details of a story I was relating. I imagined I had been overstimulated (and emotional) with the class. I had waited for a couple of weeks before I told the students about my stroke. They seemed to take it well. Maybe more than I did. The classes were all practice to me. It was the experience I needed.

My next opportunity to speak again was at a state conference on career development in the summer of 2013. I had spoken to the group before my stroke, so I hoped they would be kind to me. I told the association president about my stroke. I told him I needed to practice. I told him I wasn't "perfect." But I wanted to make sure it wouldn't be a huge embarrassment. He was happy I was getting better. He invited me to speak and use it as practice.

I prepared hard for my speech. I made slides with accompanying explanations. I practiced speaking at home. I prepared 55 slides for a 60-minute presentation.

What I didn't realize was I had created a public speaking monster. I didn't know it at the time, but it was a perfect example of executive function issues.

I thought I could do it. I had about 75 people in the audience, including the president. I knew I was in trouble as soon as I started talking. I was so scared and disorganized. Within minutes I knew I had to find a way out. There were too many slides. Time was coming to an end with fewer than half of the slides completed. With minutes to go, I told the audience about my stroke (it wasn't the topic that day) to assuage my guilt. I was disappointed and cursed out loud (I am sorry to say). I left angry and sad. I told myself I wouldn't do it again until I was really ready. I started speaking regularly in late 2014, and so far I haven't embarrassed myself!

CHAPTER ELEVEN
USE IT AND IMPROVE IT

The improvement of understanding is for two ends: first, our own increase of knowledge; secondly, to enable us to deliver that knowledge to others.

—John Locke

I had been reading about speech therapy and new treatments for aphasia. I found a lot about enriched environments—but only for rats and mice. There are not many articles about an enriched environment as a treatment for humans. The more I learned about mice, rats, and their environment, the more I understood how our (human) environment can provide the enriched components of what makes our environment fertile for improvement.

The easiest way to appreciate how an enriched environment works for mice is to look at these cages.

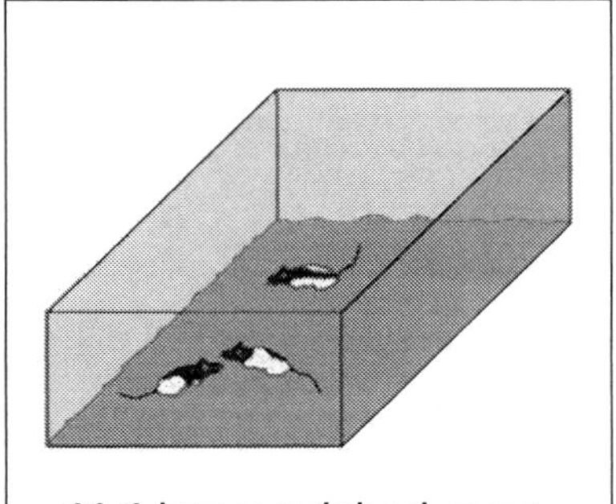

11-1 Impoverished cage.

The cage to the right (figure 11-1) is simple. There are a few mice with nothing to do. It is small and it is what the scientists call *impoverished*.

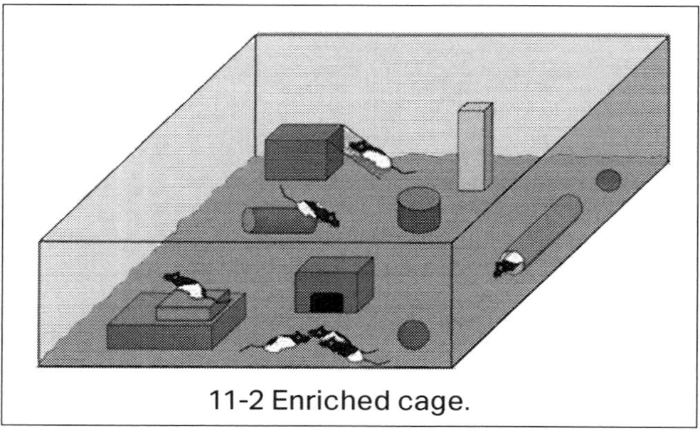

11-2 Enriched cage.

The cage above (figure 11-2) is much larger. There are lots of things to do. I imagine the mice enjoyed themselves. It looks like fun to me.

The enriched environments involved complex activities, social interaction, and novel (new, different, unusual, unique) techniques. Looking at these rodents, you can see the difference between one living quarters and another. The mice in the impoverished cage (11-1) are without toys (objects, potential stimulation). There is nothing to look at, so they likely don't do much. The mice in the enriched cage above (11-2) are clearly active, curious, and social. From my view, I'd say the rats in the impoverished cage (11-1) look sad and the ones in the enriched cage (11-2) look happy.

A rat that undergoes training can increase the number and density of synapses, dendrite length, and synapse size (Raymer). Enriched environments for rodents include cages with lots of objects (of different sizes), chains, swings, and running wheels. Many of the items were changed regularly. New sizes, new colors, new arrangements all contributed to an enriched environment. The rats were curious, probing, inquisitive, prying, and nosey. They enjoyed new tasks. Their brains were "happy" using an enriched environment, including a rotating pole (Raymer).

These tasks fit the definition of an enriched environment. The enriched (as opposed to impoverished) environment enabled plasticity to change the brain, and these changes were brought about through one experience (or task) or another.

It is difficult for a human environment *not* to be enriched. If people with aphasia live alone, have restricted social activities, are unmotivated, inactive, or just watch TV, their improvement could be stunted.

At the time, I did not understand that a difference in the environment would provide—and sometimes not—the neural improvements the environment enabled. It was my habit to live in an enriched environment. Even though my skills to communicate were damaged, my habits acted as if I wasn't damaged at all. By the time I realized the language *was* damaged, my habit had taken over. Also, I didn't realize that the act of practicing (whether I knew it or not) would further improve my "happy" brain.

I got better without knowing I was an actor in a play with an enriched environmental script. I wrote repetitively, read intensively, spoke convincingly, and listened attentively. I didn't realize it wasn't enough to write, read, speak, and listen. There was an *active* component to the play. The *active* ingredients included writing *repetitively*, reading *intensively*, speaking *convincingly*, and listening *attentively*. The beginning of the story is the same as the end: motivation and practice, practice, practice. I practiced reading, writing, and speaking without knowing that practice was all that was needed. I used it and improved it.

CHAPTER TWELVE

SPECIFICITY

No problem can be solved until it is reduced to some simple form. The changing of a vague difficulty into a specific, concrete form is a very essential element in thinking.

—J. P. Morgan

I had never heard about "working memory" before. It didn't even show up as a deficit in my deficit world of aphasia. I had some problems with memory issues. They were small in comparison to the reading and writing deficits. They were so small I didn't even notice until I experienced a new (and now visible) deficit. Working memory stores information for (almost) immediate use. It has to be recorded, accessed, and "played back" straightaway with new information that has just arrived (Cowan). People with aphasia often have working memory deficits affecting language (Wright).

The new problem started right after we moved to Florida. I had signed up as a volunteer at the local hospital in St. Augustine. My position was "patient transporter." We used wheelchairs and took patients in and out of the hospital (and sometimes within the hospital). We signed in every day with our personal code and a pager. When the pager rang, we called in to the switchboard (the computer, really), and it told us the name, room number, and destination of a patient. It was all done by computer.

The voice messages did not pronounce the first and last names out loud. It said the names of the patient, one letter at a time. So instead of a voice message that said two words, "Tom Broussard," it used 12 letters individually to say, "B-R-O-U-S-S-A-R-D, T-O-M."

When I first accessed this system, my volunteer partner was looking over my shoulder. That was the beginning. He pointed at my notes and said, "What is that?" I was angry because this had never happened before. I (apparently) couldn't write the letters down fast enough to capture them all. I could get as far as the first two or three letters, and not hear the rest. Then the first name would start and I would jump over to it. In much the same way, I got as far as the first two or three letters and that was it.

My partner was agitated about what had happened too. I had not told him about my stroke or aphasia. He was worried. And I certainly didn't tell him about *this* particular problem because I had never experienced it.

There was one more step in the procedure. The pager rang again and provided all the info again, but in word form. So, with my own eyes, I could see and (more importantly) understand the name and room number of my patients.

I explained my stroke generally (and this specific issue) to my partner. It was his first time seeing a stroke survivor in real life. We were both worried about being able to work there ... until we realized the pager saved me.

Starting that day, I recorded each "call slip," writing as best as I could. I practiced writing the name of each slip on the top of the page. At the bottom I wrote the results from the pager. Then I compared the two.

Here are some examples (the names are fictitious):

2012

At the top of this slip, I wrote:
"B-R-U-F-/-/-/-/, M-L-L-/-/-/"
At the bottom, from my pager, I wrote:
"B-O-N-A-F-R-E-D, M-I-L-L-Y."

At the top of this slip, I wrote:
"D-E-D-D-Y, B-A-S-T-E-L-/-/-/."
At the bottom, from my pager, I wrote:
"D-E-N-N-E-E, B-A-R-B-A-R-A."

At the top of this slip, I wrote:
"Z-O-G-E-R, J-O-H-S/."
At the bottom, from my pager, I wrote:
"V-O-G-E-N, J-O-H-N."

2013

At the top of this slip, I wrote:
"M-I-M-C-K-/-/-/S-K-I, M-A-R-N-/-/-/."
At the bottom, from my pager, I wrote:
"M-I-N-C-K-I-E-C-Z, M-A-N-R-L-O-N-E."

At the top of this slip, I wrote:
"B-O-L-I-/-/-/, A-L-/-/-/."
At the bottom, from my pager, I wrote,
"B-O-N-O-N-I, A-L-D-O."

2014

At the top of this slip, I wrote:
"T-A-R-I-C-K, B-R-I-N-N-I."
At the bottom, from my pager, I wrote:
"P-A-R-K-E-R, T-R-I-N-A."

At the top of this slip, I wrote:
"S-Y-M-/-/-/, B-O-N-N-A."
At the bottom, from my pager, I wrote:
"S-N-Y-D-E-R, T-O-M-M-Y."

2015 (Before my second stroke)

At the top of this slip, I wrote:
"A-B-B-A-I-R, Z-I-O-L-E."
At the bottom, from my pager, I wrote:
"A-D-D-A-R-E, V-I-O-L-E-T."

At the top of this slip, I wrote:
"S-L-E-N-P, B-A-V-R-I-D."
At the bottom, from my pager, I wrote:
"S-L-E-M-N-P, R-A-V-I-D."

I practiced working on this for over three years. I was getting better. I could write more of the names as time went by. There were still some misspelled names, but most of them were spelled correctly.

Then I had another stroke.

Actually, I had two more TIAs (transient ischemic attacks) on July 31, 2015. I was in the hospital (the same hospital where I volunteered) for six days. I had surgery for a carotid endarterectomy (cleaning out the neck arteries) on one side. Six months later I had the other one done.

I had some problems with my language as a result of the TIAs. I used my diary again. I could write, but my handwriting was jagged and crooked. The deficits were transient and cleared up within two weeks.

I worked at the hospital again in a month. I wanted to see how my working memory was doing. It turned out that the working memory improvements I had built up over three years were damaged again. Like pond ice that forms early in the season, it can barely support its own weight. That was the case with my working memory. It didn't take much to crack it.

2015 (*After* my second stroke)

At the top of this slip, I wrote:
"B-R-/-/-F, I-R-T-/-/."
At the bottom, from my pager, I wrote:
"B-E-M-P-S, I-R-E-N-E."

At the top of this slip, I wrote:
"B-L-/-/-/, M-A-R-/-/."
At the bottom, from my pager, I wrote:
"B-L-A-N-K, M-A-R-V-I-N."

At the top of this slip, I wrote:
"H-I-/-/-/-/-/-/, R-I-/-/-/."
At the bottom, from my pager, I wrote:
"H-I-G-H-W-R-I-T-H, R-A-B-O-N."

This particular deficit was an interesting one. For one thing, it had never appeared on the radar prior to arriving in Florida. Not having seen it before, it was a deficit I couldn't see. You can't address something that doesn't exist.

The neurological capacity of working memory had been damaged along with the other deficits. The symptoms of my working memory deficits must have been masked by the other, more prominent, deficits. I can now attack the problem of this specific deficit. I am still a volunteer at the hospital. Every day, I reviewed my working memory problems with the symptoms I could now see. It was a narrow deficit needing a "very particular set of skills" (as actor Liam Neeson has said).

If I didn't have those particular skills, I would not have been able to experience (see, notice, take note, appreciate) the symptoms. I was glad I came across this deficit so that I could keep track of my symptoms, create the needed feedback, and allow awareness to increase.

CHAPTER THIRTEEN
REPETITION MATTERS

One needs but to say that, in the case of an unfamiliar sequence of syllables, only about seven can be grasped in one act, but that with frequent repetition and gradually increasing familiarity with the series this capacity of consciousness may be increased.

—Hermann Ebbinghaus

As my formal therapy unfolded, repetition and word finding were the gist of my treatment. Like any kind of practice, such as school, sports, or hobby activities, repetition seemed to be the key. "Say, do, repeat" is the general mantra. Most of the exercises (with pictures, fill-in-the-blank, lists, questions, numbers, letters, etc.) were simple, at the elementary level. I realized that my exercises looked a lot like repeated elementary school classwork. Here are some examples where repetition matters.

Word Finding

My therapist explained word-finding exercises on my first day. I knew there were plenty of words I couldn't "find" even before my therapy. When I was still at the hospital there were words I could not say. It was the beginning of understanding that *not* being able to find a word was one of the first deficits of aphasia.

The word-finding strategies included using gestures, drawing pictures, and using fill-in-the-blank sentences. If you couldn't say the word you wanted (but you could still see it in your mind), you could describe the item with other associated words. You could see yourself painting, or driving, or golfing, to help explain the activities. Visualize what you were doing and describe it in detail: color, size, shape, etc. What were you painting? A house, a person, or a landscape? What were you driving? An SUV or a convertible? Were you driving your golf cart? Or lugging your bag?

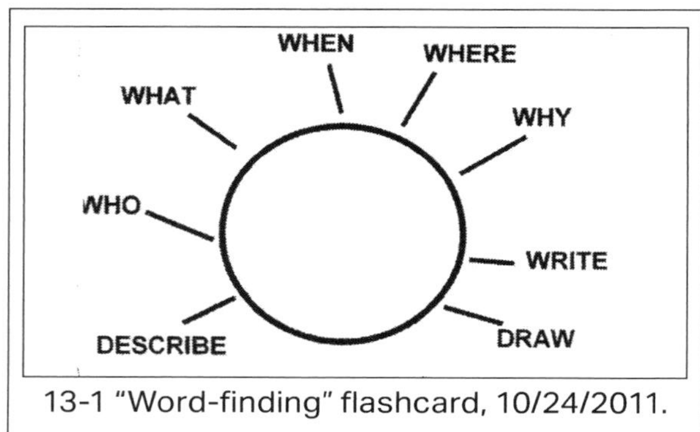

13-1 "Word-finding" flashcard, 10/24/2011.

I drew a picture (and added it in my computer) (figure 13-1): a circle in the middle of a page and the questions circling around it. I enjoyed the exercise and got many of them right. When I couldn't get them right, I used other words in the neighborhood. I meant to say "brush" and used "paint." I wanted to say "ruler" and used "screw." I wanted to say "screwdriver" and used "slot." I wanted to say "lamp" and used "light night."

As I thought about the problem, I would close my eyes (I still do this) and *think* about the item. Somehow it was a lot easier with my eyes closed, to imagine it. When I could see it (yet still couldn't say it), I *knew* what it was. I could see it in some detail. That was part of the problem and the solution.

While I was still at the hospital, I couldn't say the word "skyscraper." Even though I couldn't articulate the word, there were some parts of it (windows, bricks, lights) I could say. I got the feeling that the details were closer in my mind than the building itself. As I thought about the concept of being closer versus being farther away, it appeared to be easier (I could say the word "bricks"), rather than something more complicated (like a skyscraper). That's the way it felt to *me*.

Every time I attempted a word (that looked a lot like a nonword), it felt like it was getting closer (meaning, not as far away) to being said properly. I could *feel* the pressure of the *effort* (of thinking) that went into formulating (preparing, priming, grooming) the construction of that word.

When I couldn't find a word, it felt like a bridge leading to the word had been burned. I could see the word on the other side of the river, so to speak. I couldn't cross. I could get there (eventually) by looking for other (less complicated) bridges. Some paths brought me closer to my target. I could say other words, like "tall" and "building," but not "skyscraper." Skyscraper was a bridge too far. Some bridges were still too complicated to find my way back to my vocabulary. So I walked upriver looking for the headwaters of that particular stream of thought. When I looked back, the word always appeared closer. Somehow the repetition of the target word (and other related words) all seemed to contribute to an easier path downstream.

Long Words – Hypothermesthesias

I've always had problems with longer words. (I still do.) There was nothing magic about this. Every time I came across a long word I couldn't pronounce, I wrote it down. I wrote it in my calendar. I wrote it on 3" x 5" cards. I wrote it in my emails. I wrote it everywhere I could. That's not to say that I didn't still forget it! It requires more motivation and discipline than you can imagine. I had to repeat it over and over. Even the first syllable, *hypo*, was difficult to remember. I mapped out some connections between my target word and me. Even if I can't remember the exact word and its pronunciation (including the word, *pronunciation*), I could contact the word (like contacting the dead) through some other, more physical, connection.

After my second stroke, I had some physical defects from that as well. One of them was something called *hypothermesthesias*. It is a decreased sensitivity to heat and cold. Basically, I can't tell the difference between hot and cold in my right hand. I could not tell if the water was scalding (or if it was a hot pan) or not. That happened once or twice before I realized I had to use my other hand until I was sure about the temperature. This condition of my right hand (and somewhat, my right foot) stemmed from my TIA in the left side of my brain.

I was not aware of this problem. While I was in the hospital I felt like I was freezing. My right hand and foot were especially cold. I asked for warm sheets, but my right hand was still extremely cold. No one seemed to be worried. I continued to tell my wife about the problem with my hand feeling cold and numb. I was also dropping things—which is never fun.

An intern (doctor) came into the room on my last day there. He was very kind and appreciative of the problems with my hand. He explained about hypothermesthesias and left the room. I was discharged that day. When I got home, I had no idea about that word. I couldn't even remember the first letter of the word. I certainly didn't know the intern's name either.

After I got better I went back to my volunteer position at the hospital. I told my friends about my hot/cold problem, but no one had ever heard about it. One day while eating lunch I saw the intern leaving the cafeteria. I ran as fast as I could and grabbed him. I explained who I was, and he remembered me. I asked him again about my hot/cold issues. He answered again with hypothermesthesias. I asked him if he could write it down for me, and he did. It turned out it was his *last* day at the hospital. He was moving to a new rotation at a hospital in the Midwest. I would never have heard about this word again if I hadn't seen him that day. It's a big word for "a small world" experience.

I had seen the intern briefly and still remembered him. Clearly, it was a memorable exchange that was stored and retrieved. I couldn't remember the word, but his face was connected to it and I could remember *that*. Since then, I have printed out the word and added it to my calendar. I still cannot pronounce the word spontaneously. But I can work through it regularly (in my calendar and in my folder) to repeat it.

I recognized the face of the intern in an instant. Even though I could not say or pronounce the word, I was connected to the word through his face. Without my even knowing it, that particular memory was embedded (probably because of the emotion from my stroke) deep within my brain. The memory-event didn't sit there on the side of the road with nowhere to go. Every appropriate change in the brain is used (and matched) by plasticity.

Long Words – Melodious

I had worked at the Heller School at Brandeis University for several years. After my stroke, there were several people whose names I could not remember. That's always a problem and usually an embarrassment. I would be speaking for the first time at Heller about my stroke and aphasia. There were several people I knew but could not remember their names. I was getting used to having that problem. So if I'm going to speak at a presentation, I usually list all the people who are organizing the event, add the names to emails, and take pictures of the nameplates on their offices, or their nametags. I'd do everything I could to help connect names with faces and then remember them. It seems there are clues in everything. The brain can quickly build the structure of remembering, no matter how small.

After the presentation at Heller I went around the building looking for friends to visit. Apparently I laugh a lot, and loud. So, several friends heard me laughing. It was wonderful to see them. I still had to check their nameplate (surreptitiously)—(Wow, check out *that* word! Spell-check always helps)—to say their first name. As I mentioned, it is always a letdown if I forget a name, especially that of a good friend. Of course, many of these people are friends I had not seen for a couple of years. It is still a disappointment if I can't remember their name.

As I made my way from room to room, I came to a room with my friend who said she had heard my "melodious voice." I had not heard that word for a long time, certainly long before my stroke. I liked the word and explained to her about not being able to find certain words, especially long words like *melodious*. I told her I'd try to remember it. In her next email, Sharra signed it with "Melodiously yours." I knew that *that* word would always be connected to her name and face. I asked her to send me the story. Here it is.

> *That's great that you want to share my note on your site! So do you remember how we introduced "melodious" into our conversation? I heard you in the hallway and then you appeared at the door of my office. I immediately greeted you with a big smile and hug and said, "I thought I heard your melodious voice." That's how it all happened.*

The memory is an amazing thing. Now when I email Sharra, I am always aware of (and repeat) the connection of a name and a face linked by a long, impossible word for me to pronounce—except, now I can. It is all based on another long and impossible-to-pronounce set of words, *experience-dependent neural plasticity.*

Short Words – Acronyms

I know it sounds crazy: Using words with only three letters that aren't even words can still be a challenge. When I had my stroke, I was standing outside of our local CVS. It was on Harvard Street in Waltham, across the street from Hannaford supermarket. Laura and I walked to and from our apartment to either CVS or Hannaford almost every day for five years. This CVS is open 24/7 and has a big parking lot and customers day and night. My stroke happened in the front of the CVS and Laura dragged me into it. The CVS pharmacist called 911. The ambulance came to CVS, stabilized me in the store, and then took me out in a gurney in minutes. CVS is a large part of my life, being part of the stroke and all. Why couldn't I say the word, *CVS*, for months afterward?

The ambulance took me to MGH where I had been many times. MGH was the hospital where I had my heart surgery. MGH is the best hospital in the country, especially for cardiovascular medicine. My operation at MGH was three months before my stroke. I was discharged a week after the surgery, had visited MGH many times, and had spoken with doctors and nurses weekly. MGH is a wonderful place. Yet, I could not say the word, *MGH*, for months. Interesting: I could not spell the word, *hospital*, even one year later.

I *can* spell *tPA* these days (although saying *tissue plasminogen activator* may take more time!). One day, months later, I had to fill out an insurance form. They asked for my college degrees. It was a perfect case of "seeing it but not saying it." I got my Ph.D. five years ago, after six years of working on it. That makes 11 years of living as a *Ph.D.* without being able to say it for months. After my stroke at *CVS*, surgery at *MGH,* and treatment by *tPA*, why no three-letter words in my lexicon?

By the way, when submitting my taxes the next year, the word *IRS* seemed to be working just fine. Hmmm ... I wonder why.

CHAPTER FOURTEEN

INTENSITY MATTERS

A little each day is enough, as long as a little is produced each day.

—Payot, a friend of Santiago Ramón y Cajal

Intensive treatment simply means more therapy. Typical speech therapy usually provides about two hours a week. My SLP provided a total of 30 45-minute sessions. Within weeks, I asked my therapist if there was anything else I could do to get better. Two hours a week was a start, but it wasn't enough. She recommended an intensive therapy program in Chicago. I checked it out online. It included four to six weeks of intensive (30 hours/week) therapy of reading, writing, and speaking. It looked like an intensive program I might like. But it was too expensive. My insurance had paid for the 30 sessions. They couldn't pay for the additional intensive therapy in Chicago. But by then I was already embarking on my own accidental therapy. I spent the rest of every week trying to explain to myself what was wrong with me.

For the first couple of weeks, I had nothing to do but think. I thought about lessons which could help me understand my deficits, using metaphors and my own life stories. I couldn't write. My grammar was gone. But I used metaphorical drawings that allowed me to understand more of what I was thinking. One metaphor led me to appreciate there was more to speech therapy than two short sessions per week. I didn't make a conscious decision about one kind of treatment or another. I had enough time. So it seemed like practice (of any kind) was the right thing to do.

Full-Time *Therapeutic* Equivalent (FTTE)

At the start of my therapy, I assumed there was a one-and-only activity between the treatment and the disease (damage, impairment, injury). I received my treatment twice a week from my therapist. My disease was aphasia. Treatment included fill-in-the-blank word exercises, word-finding exercises, and sheets of repeated words. I did similar homework after each session. There was only one kind of treatment. My sessions were the highlight of the week. After a bit, they were the *only* highlight. There was only one tool. As they say, when all you have is a hammer, everything starts to look like a nail.

New tools emerged. I walked to think. I kept track with my diary. I recorded my voice to discover what was wrong. I took pictures to help me understand the world around me. The treatment was no longer a monopoly. It was no longer a one-size-fits-all therapy.

I remembered a term called "full-time equivalent" (FTE) in business, and used it as a metaphor in my diary. It is a unit that indicates the workload of a worker across similar contexts. FTE is used to measure the work of one employee. FTE of 1.0 means the person is equivalent to a full-time worker. FTE of 0.5 means the worker is a half-time worker.

I extended the metaphor. A full-time *therapeutic* equivalent (FTTE) provided a full-time share of therapy for any one patient. That was my idea, anyway. Any treatment can be used, up to one FTTE.

At the beginning, speech therapy provided one FTTE. It was my one therapy, my only treatment. The available "therapeutic space" was spent in speech therapy. That wasn't to say that all the available space was consumed. There weren't any other therapies in the corral. But the composition of the herd had begun to change. There was still just one FTTE, but additional homemade treatments found their way into the mix. The new modalities and tools crowded out speech therapy.

I don't mean I gave speech therapy short shrift. At the beginning, the only thing I knew (therapeutically speaking) was word finding and repetition. That was it. Once I started using additional treatments, there was a lot more to do. When you start with a light load of 10 credit hours and find out you need 24 credit hours to graduate, things can get intense. Speech therapy used 100 percent of the entire pie chart, and then 50 percent, and then 25 percent, and then 10 percent as other modalities assumed the load.

What had appeared as a single treatment started to separate. It didn't look like a nail anymore. FTTE was no longer relegated to one therapy or treatment. A lonely stint of speech therapy had new friends. FTTE reassembled with a number of diverse treatments, including walking, thinking, problem solving, keeping track, and feedback.

One treatment, called *speech therapy*, wasn't enough. There wasn't enough activity. The help that speech therapy did offer didn't provide the intensive, enriched energy needed to attack the problems. New treatments provided different perspectives. Different perspectives provided a new view of the deficits. By definition, experience-dependent plasticity requires the experience component of it. The more the activities, the more plasticity occurs. Limited treatment (including scant speech therapy) limits plasticity. Expansive treatment (of almost any kind) intensifies plasticity. New and more treatments are more intensive. Learning is provided by every experience. The more intensive the treatment, the more learning occurs. Every treatment (dose, prescription, remedy) that yields more improvement provides a concomitant neural structure that supports the improvement. That's the way plasticity works.

Every improvement in memory and language production comes as a result of changes in the brain. The more the doses, the more the learning. The more the learning, the more the brain changes. Every transaction (treatment, step, operation) provides a neurological step closer to awareness.

The brain can notice deficits. And the more the brain can notice the deficits, the more the brain gets closer to understanding (and resolving) the deficits. I wasn't consciously aware of creating intensive treatments per se. But therapeutic space was available and nature took its course.

CHAPTER FIFTEEN
SALIENCE MATTERS

A thing is important if anyone 'think' it important.
—William James

The salience of an idea, thought, or activity helps an individual assess large amounts of information by importance, and gives their attention to that which is ranked most important. The more salient the activity, the greater the likelihood that plasticity will be prompted. The personal relevance (salience) of one experience or another can influence the outcome (Raymer).

I didn't know much about what salience meant in terms of my aphasia. I didn't invent some idea or activity that would make the experience more salient. I experienced things that were relevant to me. It was only later I learned about the principles of plasticity and the signs indicating I was getting better *based* on plasticity and the experience-dependent principles underlying it. If I was interested (or curious) about one thought or another, it prompted a neurological spike in neural activity as a result.

Before my stroke, I had wanted to write a book. I worked in workforce development to help people with leadership and their careers. The only book I had written so far was my dissertation. I also had started a draft a long time ago, called

The Leader Within. I was writing while I was traveling to Malaysia. I was there for a month, so I figured I had plenty of time. On my way back home I stopped in Atlanta and had time to look at the newsstand. While perusing the books, I came across a book with the *exact same* title, *The Leader Within.* I couldn't believe it. I didn't know you could have books with the same title. I bought it to see if it was possible. By the time I returned home, I had read enough to know the premises of my draft and the other book were completely different, and with a different subtitle.

I never did publish my version of *The Leader Within*, but I did save it. My draft provided plenty of career ideas at Career Prospects, Inc. (my first company). I used it for articles, presentations, and company courses with the theme of careers and jobs. I had lost jobs in my life. So writing that book and starting the company were about changing and re-creating skills to prepare for a new career. I kept the other book, as well. Even though I didn't particularly like it, I kept it next to my draft.

As years went by, I got my Ph.D., closed my company (after 15 years), and took a new job at the university, where I got my doctorate. The topic of my research degree continued to be workforce development. Soon after graduating, I got a new job as Assistant (and then Associate) Dean, Admissions & Career Services. I enjoyed my work in admissions and career services. It was a new job and there was plenty of time for me to explore what the next stage might look like.

Then I had my stroke.

This ended my career in workforce development. Or so I thought. As I started my therapy and researched my new skills, I had a new thought. I couldn't read, write, or speak well, but I discovered my thinking wasn't damaged (at least, that's what they told me). As I gathered the records from my rehabilitation, I thought about writing a new book.

For decades I had been thinking about writing the earlier book. I must have talked about my goals, including writing a book, with my therapist and my doctor. In their own notes, both of them mentioned my idea of "writing a book." It activated my recovery through the salient (noticeable, important, obvious) idea of writing my book. I always wanted to write a book. Now all I had to do was actually *fix* my writing and then I could *write* any book.

As I've mentioned, the only book I had written before my stroke was my dissertation. Even though it wasn't a *real* book, I held it up as an example of what I could do. The title of my dissertation was: "Who Is Accommodating Whom? Small Business Practices and Attitudes regarding Hiring People with Disabilities: An Exploratory Study." How ironic. I had done a lot of work with people with disabilities and their careers. If ever there was a vested interest in disability studies, my stroke brought it home. My stroke was the ultimate pink slip. Writing about disability and losing one's career is as salient as can be.

CONCLUSION

ENRICHED SPEECH THERAPY

I was a successful experiment, but an experiment nonetheless. I got better, but we are still not sure how it happened. I received all the therapy my insurance afforded me. That included 30 hours of speech therapy and 22 hours of aphasia group therapy. Those 50 some-odd hours were spread across six months of treatment.

But here is the question. Did I get better as a result of those 50 hours of speech therapy? We will never know. And we will never know because the 50 hours of *outside* therapy were tossed in among the 1,700 hours of my own *intensive* therapy.

Learning what I have learned about aphasia recovery, I can say the difference between 50 hours and 1,700 hours is stark. A few hours with a professional speech therapist definitely provide a good start. However, recovery needs more than what speech therapy alone can offer. The cost and insurance factors can be part of the solution. If more stroke survivors were to be admitted into intensive programs, that could help. More resources from insurance companies means more therapist hours (also in intensive programs) for the patient. Still, you're left with a paltry sum of hours, compared to a new configuration of recovery.

The current (clinical) thoughts about recovery are established like a school. There is one class with one teacher and one student. The student goes to class twice a week. That's it. The student attends with some idea that these classes can help. And there is some homework. But not enough to sustain the flow of thinking from one week (or one class) to another. There is no curriculum such that you can "look ahead" and see what else has to be studied.

What has to change is an understanding that there is a larger context of recovery, with a lot more moving parts than just speech therapy. Again using a school metaphor, a college degree takes four years. As a stroke survivor student, you get a small amount of "learning" (from your teacher) and then it is over. And you are still stuck as a freshman. You have three and a half years to go with no curriculum, no classes, and no teachers. In addition, there will be no degree. The concept of recovery (or graduation) doesn't exist, other than completing the only class which you have been assigned. That is the problem.

This new context of recovery changes the idea of how a person with aphasia learns. A person with aphasia learns from experiences on the inside. A successful student might appear to be learning from a great teacher. And that can be the case for some teachers and students willing to be taught. But it is different for people (or students) with aphasia. For one thing, a person with aphasia will have a hard time being taught when "being taught" is part of the problem. What little information is provided will dissolve into an ocean of unknown needs. The only thing that an aphasic can do is learn. And most of the learning is accomplished below the surface.

All brains learn all the time, whether awake or asleep. The structure of the organ is designed that way. The brain works hard while awake and consolidates many frayed threads while asleep. Food provides the needs of the body. Thinking provides the needs of the brain. Short and intermittent therapy does not provide the needs required. Lifelong learning provides sustenance to long-term recovery. It is a critical element of rehabilitation. It isn't enough to attend SLP sessions *as if* the sessions will provide all the learning and, as a result, all the energy. SLP sessions must be refashioned with a full understanding of how the brain learns from sustainable, persistent experience. There is a bright future of continuous improvement if the learning activities are also continuous.

The task of each therapy session should not be just about identifying the proper response, such as remembering a name or spelling a word or identifying an object in a picture. It isn't good enough to answer a canned set of questions correctly. It is more than that. Understanding the underlying process of being *aware* of the deficits is the core of learning. Therapy sessions provide a narrow view of the process. Having said that, speech therapy is still incredibly valuable. Speech therapy orients the start of your therapeutic life. After the classes end, though, the need for more therapy is still needed. That is the issue. For most aphasics, those few classes typically can't provide the momentum required to launch a multiyear effort of learning.

It has been almost five years since my stroke and my stroke was relatively mild. My aphasia left me unable to read, write, and speak well for almost a year. The next two years were spent working on my ability to read and write well. And another year provided more writing and public speaking. People ask me all the time if I am fully healed. I appear to be "perfect" in their eyes. I tell people that I am doing very well. But I am by no means "perfect." I am just able to "fake" my way along with the remaining aphasia symptoms.

I acquired the therapeutic momentum as a result of accidental activities that created the enriched environment I now espouse. There is a real difference between conventional therapy and enriched therapy, and it is more a shift in the approach to recovery. The context of recovery is based on time. The perspective of a therapist is short term, data driven, budget aware, and objective. The perspective of a patient is almost unknown, pending more awareness and improvement. As a result it is a race between one's perspective and another. The therapist knows, regardless of improvement, that they will part company when the contract ends. And regardless of awareness or improvement, the patient is still only starting on a long journey of recovery.

This is where the rubber meets to road. The sessions were wonderful in their own way. But they were over. And it was time to start a new stage of learning. And if "learning how to learn" wasn't part of the previous lessons, you and your family are on your own.

The speech therapy profession must convert the idea of recovery into the ethic of "learning how to learn." Every therapy day must be converted into an "every day is a *session* day" mentality. The day comes too quickly when the conventional therapy sessions end. And without a long-term plan for continued activity and improvement, the little momentum that had been started will wane.

The brain needs to exercise every day. And it can't sit by and wait for someone else to tell you what to do. The brain works by being engaged. It creates a mental tension that allows the ebb and flow of thought to arise. Problem solving without the problem doesn't provide the hook. The sessions have to be constructed to allow a future to be considered.

This future won't exist without an overarching context of recovery over and above the sessions allowed by insurance. For me, each session had its own beginning, middle, and end. There was no discussion of the future or what would happen after the therapy was over. There was no discussion of additional long-term tasks to be considered on a week-to-week or month-to-month basis. The tasks were limited to the exercises in the playbook. Nothing went beyond that. I began to wonder if there was another world outside of my scripted reality. It turned out to be the same world and the same reality. But my efforts were only scripted—if I had not confronted the reality of needing to do more *doing*.

Therapists provide the basics of recovery: automatics, word finding, and repetition. Therapists can help only up to a point. Counterintuitively, part of the point of speech therapy is to withdraw the aid. The electric starter in a car engages, but not until the engine kicks in. A therapist cannot be engaged *on behalf* of the person who needs to be engaged. A therapist cannot be motivated *on behalf* of the person who needs to be motivated. The only thing a therapist can do is provide the scaffolding of the structure yet to come. The enriched environment provides the support, but it can't be imported. It has to be organically grown. The seed bed must be sowed from the beginning. Waiting until the end of speech therapy sessions to begin the next stage is too late. Tilling and amending the soil is needed long before planting the seeds.

The transition from *conventional* speech therapy to *enriched* speech therapy requires more therapeutic energy. In the absence of a speech therapist in residence, *enriched* therapy requires regular, persistent, *personal* therapy. The mission of speech therapists is to help people with aphasia understand the overarching context of recovery: It is a marathon, not a sprint. Every day is a session day, whether you are seeing the therapist, walking around town, or writing in your diary. Re-creating one's language requires a continuous loop of activity, evidence, and feedback.

It has become clear in the literature that aphasia gets better from therapy and substantially better from intensive therapy (Kleim). Enriched therapy is intensive. The difference is that enriched therapy represents an ethic of learning in the absence of any external teaching resources. Enriched therapy isn't looking for the right or wrong responses as much as it must *experience* the responses and look for what grows.

Word finding and repetition were the start with conventional speech therapy. Intensive speech therapy provides more therapeutic hours, but still woefully fewer hours than what enriched therapy requires.

The new, enriched elements of speech therapy provide an enhanced atmosphere of learning far beyond one exercise or another. Speech therapy needs to transition to an enriched therapeutic culture that includes the long-term therapeutic responsibility for speech-language pathology. The responsibility of the therapist is to create tasks that encourage *more tasks to be assigned* by the patient.

The secret of aphasia recovery is about the *doing*, and synaptic connections are the key. Those connections deliver the ever increasing learning field. It is in our nature; the brain *wants* to build more networks. More experience, more practice, more variety, and more *life* provide the learning. Experience-dependent neural plasticity is the master builder. Enriched speech therapy provides the missing link.

GLOSSARY

aphasia – The loss of the ability to read, write, or speak, or understand spoken or written language due to disease or injury of the brain.

automatics – These are products of language including the alphabet, numbers, days of the week, months of the year, and time. Deficits of aphasia include not being able to say a word of an automatic set without reciting each item in the set until the right word is found.

axon – The neuron's long and unbranched fiber which carries impulses from the cell to a neighboring neuron.

Broca's area – A region of the brain located behind the left temple, which is associated with speech.

CAT scan (CT scan) – Computed tomography, more commonly known as a CT or CAT scan, is a diagnostic medical test that, like a traditional X-ray, produces multiple images or pictures of the inside of the body. CT scanning of the head is typically used to detect infarction, tumors, calcifications, hemorrhage, and bone trauma.

dendrite – The branched extension from the cell body of a neuron, which receives impulses from other neurons through synaptic contacts.

electroencephalogram (EEG) – The EEG is a test used to detect abnormalities related to electrical activity of the brain. This procedure tracks and records brain wave patterns. Small metal discs with thin wires (electrodes) are placed on the scalp, and they send signals to a computer to record the results.

emergency medical technicians (**EMTs**) – They are health-care providers or clinicians of emergency medical services. They are trained to respond quickly to emergency situations regarding medical issues, traumatic injuries, and accident scenes.

executive function – The ability to organize cognitive processes, including the ability to plan ahead, prioritize, and monitor one's own behavior.

full-time therapeutic equivalent (FTTE) – A full-time share of therapy for any one patient.

Gamma Knife® – The Gamma Knife® is used to treat brain tumors by administering high-intensity cobalt radiation therapy in a manner that concentrates the radiation over a small area. The patient wears a specialized helmet that is surgically fixed to the skull. The brain tumor remains stationary at the target point of the gamma rays.

ischemic stroke – This occurs as a result of an obstruction within a blood vessel supplying blood to the brain.

lesion – Any abnormal tissue found in an organism, often the brain, usually damaged by disease, trauma, or stroke.

magnetic resonance imaging (MRI) – A neuroimaging technique which uses magnetic energy to generate images that reveal structural details in the brain and the body.

metacognition – The process of considering and regulating one's own learning and thinking process.

neologism – Describes the use of a word that has meaning only to the person who uses it, independent of its common meaning. Neologisms may be related to aphasia acquired after brain damage resulting from a stroke or head injury.

neuron – The basic cell making up the brain and nervous system, consisting of a cell body, a long fiber (axon) that transmits impulses, and many short fibers (dendrites) that receive them. There are about 100 billion neurons in the brain, each one connecting with 1,000 to 100,000 synapses.

numeracy – The ability to reason with numbers and mathematical concepts.

occupational therapy (O/T) – O/T is the use of assessment and treatment to develop, recover, or maintain the daily living and work skills of people with a physical, mental, or cognitive disorder.

paraphasia – A symptom in aphasia which refers to the substitution of a word with a nonword that preserves at least half of the segments and/or number of syllables of the intended word, or a problem associated with aphasia and characterized by the production of unintended syllables, words, or phrases during the effort to speak.

physical therapy (PT) – PT includes therapists that help heal impairments and promote mobility, function, and quality of life through examination, diagnosis, prognosis, and physical intervention.

plasticity – The ability to change the organization of synapses and networks of neurons, based on new experiences.

pt. – patient.

scholastic assessment test (SAT) – Standardized tests widely used for college admissions in the United States of America.

semantic memory – This refers to a portion of long-term memory that processes ideas and concepts that are not drawn from personal experience. It includes things that are common knowledge, such as the names of colors, the sounds of letters, the capitals of countries, and other basic facts acquired over a lifetime.

speech-language pathologists (SLPs) – SLPs are also called speech-language therapists or speech therapists. They specialize in the evaluation and treatment of communication disorders including aphasia and swallowing disorders.

stroke – Also referred to as a cerebrovascular accident (CVA), it is the loss of brain function due to a lesion or disturbance in the blood supply to the brain. This disturbance is due to either ischemia (lack of blood flow) or hemorrhage (the flow of blood from a ruptured blood vessel). As a result, the affected area of the brain cannot function normally, which might result in an inability to move one or more limbs on one side of the body, failure to understand or formulate speech, or a vision impairment on one side of the visual field.

synapse – A structure which permits a neuron to pass an electrical or chemical signal across a small gap between one neuron cell and another. Each neuron will grow between 1,000 to 100,000 synapses. A part of the brain the size of a grain of sand would contain about 1 billion synapses.

syntax – The rules and conventions governing the order of words in phrases, clauses, and sentences.

tissue plasminogen activator (tPA) – A protein used to dissolve blood clots, to treat ischemic strokes. Typically, the drug must be administered within three hours.

transient ischemic attack (TIA) – A brief episode of cerebral ischemia that is usually characterized by temporary blurring of vision, slurring of speech, numbness, paralysis, or syncope (a spontaneous loss of consciousness), and which is often predictive of more serious cerebral accidents – also called little stroke, ministroke.

United States Secretary of the Navy (SECNAV) – The Secretary of the Navy is the head of the Department of the Navy, a military department within the Department of Defense of the United States of America.

BIBLIOGRAPHY

Brookshire R. H., "The Role of Auditory Functions in Rehabilitation of Aphasic Individuals." Veterans Administration Hospital, Minneapolis. (No date).

Caspari, I., Parkinson, S., LaPointe, L., Katz, R. "Working Memory and Aphasia." *Brain and Cognition* 37, 205–223 (1998).

Cowan, N. "Multiple Concurrent Thoughts: The Meaning and Developmental Neuropsychology of Working Memory." *Dev. Neuropsychol.* Sept. 2010; 35 (5): 447–474.

Hattie, J., and Timperley, H. "The Power of Feedback." *Review of Educational Research*, March 2007; vol. 77, no. 1, 81–112.

Immordino-Yang, M., Christodoulou, J., Singh, V. "Rest Is Not Idleness: Implications for the Brain's Default Mode for Human Development and Education." *Perspectives on Psychological Science*, 2012, 7 (4), 352–364.

James, William. *The Principles of Psychology, Volume One.* Dover Publications Inc., New York, 1918 (1890).

Kleim, J., and Jones, T. "Principles of experience-dependent neural plasticity: Implications for rehabilitation after brain damage." *Journal of Speech, Language, and Hearing Research*, 51, 225–239 (2008).

Lakoff, G., and Johnson, M. *Metaphors We Live By*. The University of Chicago Press, Chicago and London. 1980.

LeDoux, Joseph. *Synaptic Self: How Our Brains Become Who We Are.* Penguin Books. New York, 2002.

Raymer, A. et al. "Translational Research in Aphasia: From Neuroscience to Neurorehabilitation." *Journal of Speech, Language, and Hearing Research*, 51, 259–275 (2008).

Ross, Deborah, and Spencer, Sara. *Aphasia Rehabilitation: An Auditory and Verbal Task Hierarchy*. Charles C. Thomas Publisher, Springfield, IL, 1980.

Wright, H., and Fergadiotis, G. "Conceptualizing and Measuring Working Memory and Its Relationship to Aphasia." *Aphasiology*; 26 (3–4): 258–278 (2012).

NOTES

Notes

How to Contact the Author

Thomas G. Broussard, Jr., Ph.D., founder of Stroke Educator, Inc., is running a 50-state Aphasia Awareness Campaign, talking about stroke, aphasia, and recovery. If you would like Dr. Broussard to speak to your group, please contact him by telephone at 207-798-1449, e-mail at tbroussa@comcast.net, or mail addressed to Stroke Educator, Inc., 541 Domenico Circle, St. Augustine, FL 32086

Also by Thomas G. Broussard, Jr., Ph.D.

Stroke Diary: A Primer for Aphasia Therapy

www.StrokeEducator.com